Covid-19 in Palestine

Unsettling Colonialism in Our Times

The Unsettling Colonialism in Our Times series publishes books at the intersection of settler colonialism studies, decolonisation, and critiques of neoliberalism, illuminating the complex relationship between power and knowledge in the 21st Century. It encourages research which has previously been studied as 'post-colonial' or as examples of successful 'end of history' processes of modernisation and westernisation to be viewed in light of the struggles for national liberation, democracy and human rights. The series is a unique meeting point between new and established scholars who engage with activist intellectual work concerning the welfare and future of the most oppressed communities in the world.

Series Editors
William Gallois, Director of Research at the Institute of Arab and Islamic Studies
Ilan Pappe, Professor of History; and Director of the European Centre for Palestine Studies
Both at University of Exeter, UK
Advisory Board
Lorenzo Veracini, Swinburne University of Technology in Melbourne, Australia Robert J. C. Young, New York University
Eyal Weizmann, Goldsmiths Ruba Salih, SOAS
Katsuya Hirano, UCLA
Angela Woollacott, Australian National University

Covid-19 in Palestine

The Settler Colonial Context

Nadia Naser-Najjab

I.B. TAURIS

LONDON • NEW YORK • OXFORD • NEW DELHI • SYDNEY

I.B. TAURIS
Bloomsbury Publishing Plc
50 Bedford Square, London, WC1B 3DP, UK
1385 Broadway, New York, NY 10018, USA
29 Earlsfort Terrace, Dublin 2, Ireland

BLOOMSBURY, I.B. TAURIS and the I.B. Tauris logo are trademarks of
Bloomsbury Publishing Plc

First published in Great Britain 2023

Series design by Toby Way
Cover image: *The Oppressed Press* © Beesan Arafat

ISBN: HB: 978-0-7556-5116-0
PB: 978-0-7556-5117-7
ePDF: 978-0-7556-5118-4
eBook: 978-0-7556-5119-1

Typeset by Deanta Global Publishing Services, Chennai, India

To find out more about our authors and books visit www.bloomsbury.com and
sign up for our newsletters.

In memory of my beloved friend Shireen Abu Aqla, the 'voice of Palestine'. These days, I always find myself looking back on our times together, wishing you were still here.

Contents

Acknowledgements

I would first like to thank Shireen Abu Aqla, the globally renowned journalist who was my dearest friend. She contributed to this book through various conversations and a June 2021 interview that addressed the Palestinian vaccine scandal. Shireen was killed by an Israeli sniper while reporting in Jenin refugee camp on 11 May, 2022. I feel sad and angry that she did not live to see this book published.

I would like to express my deep gratitude to the book's interviewees, such as the Gazans who spoke to me during the 2021 war in the Strip, who showed their belief in my work by taking the time and effort to speak to me, often in life-threatening circumstances. I am sure the bonds and connections that we formed during these interviews will last over time and that we will work together in the future. I am thankful to artist Dr. Beesan Arafat for the cover image of the book.

I would also like to thank my editor Ben Boulton for his thorough work on the manuscript.

And finally, I would like to express my deep gratitude to my husband, Walid, and my daughters, Leen and Nadine, for their support, encouragement and understanding at all times and especially during lockdown.

Introduction

The pandemic began in Palestine in March 2020, when the first Covid-19 cases were traced back to visiting American tourists, who then isolated in the city's Hotel Angel. The Palestinian Authority (PA)[1] immediately declared a state of emergency, closed Bethlehem and imposed a lockdown. Volunteers from the city established an emergency committee that assisted residents during the lockdown, while Palestinians from the rest of the West Bank sent food, medical supplies and disinfectant. Both the prime minister and the health minister held press conferences, where they provided updates on the situation, including information about case numbers and recovery rates. The PA established various committees, including the National Emergency Committee (which includes local governors and security force heads), the Epidemiology Committee (which includes medical specialists) and the National Committee for CORONA (which includes health civil society stakeholders and NGOs), who each provided assessments and recommendations to the minister of health.

The PA was viewed increasingly favourably by the Palestinian public,[2] and representatives of international organizations praised the Palestinian government for its initial response to the pandemic,[3] despite the fact that a month after the initial outbreak, the PA had not published a pandemic plan. Elias al-Arja, the general manager of the Angel Hotel in Beit Jala, questions this acclaim. He explains:

> [The] PA could enforce law and enforce lockdown, but nothing more. [The] PA did not support us or provide anything, except for tests and transfer patients to hospital if needed. People sent food and other supplies. [The] PA imposed lockdown and Palestinian security forces enforced it. We Hotel owners took care of everything for corona cases. People also adhered to rules and took measures.

He notes the initial response began to lose momentum within one year.

> During the period of the first cases, cooperation between Hotel owner[s] and people managed the crisis of the virus very well. A year later, PA is unable to protect people and people have no confidence in PA, even to provide vaccine. PA did not compensate us for the closure during lock down. There is an approval from PM to compensate us, a budget of one and half million, but [we] have not received anything.[4] [And] when the PA 'tried to contact Israeli authorities and tourist offices and companies to find flights for the stranded tourists, it was chaos and responses took time'.

Dr Salwa Najjab expressed similar sentiments in a follow-up interview. She observes: '[When] the 4th wave of Corona hit, [the] PA took no action. [The] Covid committees [were] inactive and no awareness campaigns [were] available. No serious work [was done] on post corona issues and [there were] no vaccination[s] for children.'[5] She also refers to a WHO report that highlighted a number of weaknesses and deficiencies that have still not been addressed. It observes:

> COVID-19 has underlined the need for cross-sectoral engagement to improving population health and addressing the determinants of health inequities. The right to health for all depends on maintaining and improving essential health care, for which expanded domestic and international commitment and investment is vital. Immediate support is needed to address the critical situation jeopardizing sustained provision of referral services to Palestinian patients'.[6]

When the pandemic broke out, Palestine was already experiencing protracted economic, political and social crisis. The stagnation of the peace process, deeply rooted political divides and external political pressures weighed heavily on Palestinians, suffocating their national aspirations. The pandemic was merely the latest in a series of national catastrophes.

In the pandemic, the (already immense) gap between Israel and the territories has become a chasm. As Palestinians resort to crude survival measures, Israel has surged ahead in the global vaccination race. In mid-February 2021, almost one year after Covid-19 broke out, it was celebrated as a vaccination 'world leader'.[7] Just one month later, it came out of lockdown and began to reopen.[8] But the pandemic continued in Palestine – in February 2022, 586,355 confirmed cases and 5,181 virus-related deaths were recorded in the occupied Palestine territory (oPt),[9] and in the period 2–12 February, the Ministry of Education moved teaching online.

In an open letter to the University of Oxford, health and human rights organizations challenged the prevailing narrative that celebrates Israel's pandemic response. In it, they claimed that 'adding these millions of vaccine-deprived Palestinians to Israel's figures would change the picture entirely'.[10] With grim and entirely predictable inevitability, the Israeli government responded by alleging this criticism had 'anti-Semitic' motivations.[11]

Israel continues to deny responsibility for Palestinians who live and die under its occupation, and even non-citizen Palestinians in Israel, including one Palestinian student from the West Bank who studies at Tel Aviv University.[12] It has not imposed any movement restrictions on Jewish settlers in the West Bank and has instead upheld their freedom of movement. And it continues to fail to comply with Article 56 of the Fourth Geneva Convention and specifically its requirement to guarantee 'the adoption and application of the prophylactic and preventive measures necessary to combat the spread of contagious diseases and epidemics'. And this is why Amnesty International called on Israel to 'stop ignoring its international obligations as an occupying power and immediately ensure that Covid-19 vaccines are equally and fairly provided to Palestinians living under its occupation in the West Bank and the Gaza Strip'.[13]

Israel initially blocked the supply of Russian vaccines and claimed that under the 1994 Paris Protocol, its Ministry of Health could only allow medicines to be distributed in the oPt that had passed the necessary scientific and regulatory procedures. In February 2021, it, however, approved the distribution of 5,000 doses of this vaccine to the West Bank, of which less than half (2,000) were eventually administered to Palestinian health workers. However, it continued to withhold the distribution of 1,000 doses to the Gaza Strip, in the hope they could be used as a bargaining 'chip' for captured Israelis.[14]

A range of (international, Israeli and Palestinian) health and human rights organizations responded to these and other developments by issuing a statement in which they suggested Israel was legally obliged to vaccinate the oPt's inhabitants. They added that the PA's limited financial resources were a direct consequence of Israeli policies and urged the Israeli authorities not to deduct any of the proposed vaccination costs from the tax revenues it collects on the PA's behalf.[15]

There are (limited) precedents for Israel acting in its own interest to preserve Palestinian public health. For example, its draining of the Huleh swamps to fight a Malaria epidemic in the early 1950s was accompanied by self-serving appeals to advancing 'development' and 'modernity' (see Shavit, 2015: Chapter 2). Palestinian resistance, therefore, was viewed as being against modernity rather than the loss of livelihoods and dispossession. Settlers later incorporated these tropes into the historical narrative of Zionist pioneers 'redeeming' the land (Anton, 2008: 90).[16]

It is therefore perhaps surprising that Israel fails to take basic measures to prevent the spread of Covid-19 among the 20,000 Palestinians who work in Israel.[17] The Israeli government initially said it would vaccinate Palestinian workers with permits, failing to acknowledge the thousands who work without documentation.[18] It then suspended vaccination while citing 'administrative delays',[19] before resuming without any explanation.[20],[21]

When one Palestinian worker developed Covid-19 symptoms, he was dumped at a checkpoint near Ramallah.[22] Even after statistics demonstrated that Palestinians who worked in Israeli settlements had the second highest number of infections of any vocational group in the oPt, they were allowed to continue to work (in capsules),[23] despite ongoing lockdowns in the territories.[24]

Israel has a clear incentive to refrain from imposing restrictions or requirements on Palestinians who work in Israel because as Shay

Pauzner, the deputy director of the Israel Builders Association, observes, the 'Palestinians are the backbone of the entire industry'.[25] Even before the pandemic, these workers already had limited rights and were, in the absence of union representation, required to apply for permits or seek a different employer.[26] This was underlined in January 2021, when Pauzner's Association asked the Israeli government to vaccinate working Palestinians on their behalf. The pandemic also enabled Israel to track Palestinian workers and use surveillance technology. In citing the pretext of countering the pandemic, Israel asked workers to use phone applications that would enable it to access their data and information (Hanieh and Ziadeh, 2022: 14).[27]

Israel does not just fail to address the pandemic in Palestine but also seeks to exploit it for its own purposes. This was made clear when it provided vaccines to countries (including the Czech Republic, Guatemala, Honduras and Hungary) that recognized its claim to Jerusalem and relocated their embassies there.[28] Israel also provided the Syrian regime with vaccines after it released an Israeli woman who had, apparently by mistake, crossed into its territory.[29] And it was also made clear when Israel said it would permit vaccinated Palestinians to enter Jerusalem to pray at Al-Aqsa Mosque in the first Friday of the Ramadan period.[30] Sheikh Omar al-Kiswani, the Aqsa Mosque manager, warns that Israel is using the pretext of the pandemic to block entrance to Muslims, permit Jewish settlers to enter and also undertake excavations.[31]

Israel's 'security' operations in the West Bank also continue to disrupt and undermine Palestinian attempts to respond to the pandemic. On 5 November 2020, Israeli security forces, in implementing the annexation plan, uprooted seventy-four members of the Bedouin community (half of whom were children) in Khirbet Humsah, which is in the north of the Jordan Valley. B'Tselem observes: 'While the world deals with the coronavirus crisis, Israel has devoted time and effort to harassing Palestinians instead of helping protected residents living under its control.'[32] In East Jerusalem, Israel closed a PA virus testing clinic, leaving Palestinians to face their fate.[33] In March 2021, Israeli army raided the Palestinian Health Work Committees (HWC) and confiscated documents and hard discs.[34] In the same month, a 69-year-old woman died from a heart attack when Israeli soldiers stormed her house and began searching.[35]

The colonialization activities within Israel, which have been ongoing from the end of military rule (Sa'di, 2016),[36] have been equally disruptive – in February 2021 it demolished Al-Araqeeb village in the Naqab desert, one of fifty-one 'unrecognized villages' currently threatened by demolition, leaving residents homeless in freezing temperatures.[37] An OCHA report observes that Israel has demolished or forced Palestinians to demolish or confiscate 415 buildings in the period between the start of the pandemic and September 2020.[38] Israeli spokespersons invariably invoke feeble pretexts such as 'law enforcement' or 'building and planning considerations' in the full knowledge that Palestinians have almost no way to build legally.[39]

These dimensions of inactivity, neglect and active disruption attest to a fundamental health inequality and a broader apartheid reality. In a recent report, B'Tselem, the prominent Israeli human rights group, observes:

> In the entire area between the Mediterranean Sea and the Jordan River, the Israeli regime implements laws, practices and state violence designed to cement the supremacy of one group – Jews – over another – Palestinians. A key method in pursuing this goal is engineering space differently for each group. (B'tselem, 2021)[40]

This apartheid reality extends to the (4,400) Palestinian prisoners in Israeli prisons who continue to be denied a Covid-secure environment.[41] When the Legal Center for Arab Minority Rights (Adalah) petitioned the Israeli Supreme Court and demanded that social distancing guidelines be followed, the Court ruled 'that Palestinians held in prison are no different than family members or flatmates living in the same home'.[42] To add insult to injury, they also have to pay high military court fines for bails and canteen provision.[43] The health and well-being of child detainees are also affected by denied family visits and delayed court proceedings

(UNICEF, 2020: 7).[44] Medical Aid for Palestinians (MAP) reports on the dire process, which includes deliberate Israeli obstructions,[45] involved in transferring Palestinians to Jerusalem and Israeli hospitals for critical health cases. These restrictions arise even if they have all the required documents and permits, which leads to death in some cases.[46]

The expropriation of Palestinian homes and the destruction of Palestinian infrastructure (and water, sanitation and hygiene (WASH) infrastructure in particular) have substantially impeded Palestinian efforts to limit virus spread.[47] Under the Oslo Accords, Israel controls Palestinian water resources, which clearly limits the Palestinian ability to act in accordance with WASH best practices.

The colonial character of the pandemic was further underscored in mid-June 2021 when the PA agreed a deal with Israel that would result in it receiving 1.4 million doses of the Pfizer-BioNTech vaccine. Under the terms of the agreement, the PA would provide the same amount to Israel when it received a shipment of the same amount later in the year.[48] Palestinians erupted with anger when they learnt of the agreement. In response, Mohammad Shtayyeh, the PA prime minister, announced the cancellation of the deal and the establishment of an investigation committee. Mai Al-Kaila, the Palestinian health minister, and Hussein Al-Sheikh, the civil affairs minister, exchanged mutual accusations and tried to distance themselves from the deal. Al-Kaila alleged that Al-Sheikh had negotiated the deal with COGAT (Coordination of Government Activities in the Territories), although he denied any involvement.[49]

I interviewed Shireen Abu Akleh,[50] a journalist who attended a closed press conference held by Al-Kaila on 20 June 2021. According to Shireen, Al-Kaila told journalists that the Health Ministry directly negotiated the deal with the Israelis, with the aim of addressing a vaccine shortage in schools and universities. However, the actual vaccine expiry date was different from the one in the agreement. The PA also did not have the capacity to administer the vaccines before they expired.

In responding to rising public anger, the PA decided to cancel the deal. A number of other factors were also important: for example, the

PA rejected an Israeli request to not send any vaccines to the Gaza Strip and also took issue with the use of the 'State of Palestine' logo on headed papers (the PA eventually accepted this objection).[51] However, Israel, as the occupying power, is responsible for providing vaccinations to Palestinians. Hanan Ashrawi, a former PLO executive committee member, tweeted: 'If this isn't racism and corruption I don't know what is! Israel uses Palestine as dumping grounds for expired vaccines after having adamantly refused to supply them earlier, and then demands their replacement from Pfizer.'[52] In response, Palestinians took to the streets to protest against both the deal and the killing of a Palestinian activist by Palestinian security forces. Protesters openly challenged the PA's political authority (chanting 'The people want the fall of the regime') and called for security coordination while likening it to the collaborationist village leagues that Israel sought to establish in the late 1970s and early 1980s. Protesters also openly accused the security forces of acting against Palestinian national interests.[53]

In responding to this and broader pressure, the PA created an independent fact-finding committee and tasked it with investigating the deal. The committee released its report on 6 July, which accused Israel of practicing 'medical apartheid' and ignoring its responsibility, as an occupying power, to provide vaccinations for Palestinians. The report also criticized the Ministry of Health for signing the contract too quickly and not drawing on legal and political consultations. It also observed the Ministry did not take appropriate safety measures when handling the vaccination.[54] Dr Salwa Najjab, a member of the Independent Fact-finding Committee, told me:

> The near expired deal led to vaccine hesitancy, Palestinians do not trust Israel and there is no confidence in the Palestinian health system. Also, there was no follow up after we published our findings. People have the right to know and measures should be taken to mitigate and avoid any future mistakes. [The] lack of follow up increased vaccine hesitancy.[55]

One interviewee went further to allege that the PA wanted to profit from vaccinations, and they cited the 2020 Wakfet Izz Fund (Dignified Stand) affair in support. This is consistent with Silvia Federici's observation that the Palestinian elite or 'client' class, the product of foreign aid, has been engaged in extensive 'individual wealth accumulation' in the pandemic (Hanieh, 2016: 42).[56] It is also consistent with the claim that the PA has sought to extract the maximum political benefit from its pandemic interventions.[57]

Central argument and theoretical approach

When I first began writing this book, I wanted to examine how Palestinians sought to endure the pandemic while struggling within a settler colonial environment, and specifically in adjusting to land fragmentation, heightened internal divisions and a growing dependence on international funding. Through reading this book, I hope the reader will come to comprehend how the pandemic is effectively grafted onto pre-existent (colonial) patterns and relations.

I argue that established colonial realities in the oPt influence the ongoing pandemic in crucial respects. In demonstrating that the Palestinian Authority is unable to provide services or at least take safety measures to minimize virus spread, I propose that the absence of community solidarity and other resources is not an unfortunate feature of the current situation but is instead the direct result of Israel's colonial policies. I also attribute PA inaction in the face of the ongoing crisis to colonial strategies. The pandemic has not to this extent brought about a qualitative shift in Israeli–Palestinian relations but has instead reinforced a pre-existing colonial arrangement, including the willingness of the Palestinian leadership to accept Israel's terms (see Alfred, 2005; Fanon, 1963 and 2008: 210).[58]

The state of emergency declared by President Mahmoud Abbas on 5 March 2020, which enabled him to tighten his control over civil society and the judiciary,[59] violated Palestinian Basic Law, which functions as the de facto constitution. In other parts of the world, such actions would be viewed as an interruption or suspension of the established state of affairs. Agamben therefore refers to other countries when he observes how the pandemic has enabled governments to 'do their utmost to create a climate of panic', provoking a true 'state of exception' and producing 'severe limitations on movement and the suspension of daily life and work activities for entire regions'.[60] In the oPt, in contrast, 'exceptionalism' is conversely an established[61] principle that has underpinned governance in the post-Oslo period. Abujidi reiterates this in noting that 'Palestinian [s]tates of [e]xception entail all aspects of life – not only the juridical and legal – creating multilevels of [e]xception that perpetually destroys and regenerates itself in an extreme form' (2009: 272).[62] Abbas's efforts to control the judicial system[63] are therefore an extension of his efforts to establish a 'state'[64] that is uneven, imprecise and subordinate to the 'state of exception' and power to 'let live or to let die' that Israel has established (Foucault, 2003: 245).[65] Here unpredictability is used as a mechanism of political and social control (Falah and Flint, 2004).[66] Palestinians who remained in Israel (who lived under military rule until 1966) and Palestinian refugees also live under varying degrees of 'exceptionalism'.

The 'international community' is also deeply implicated in the persistence of this 'state'. When Mohammad Shtayyeh, the Palestinian prime minister, announced austerity and cost cutting,[67] it was made clear that the security forces, as a kind of privileged class, would be exempt, despite the fact that this would disadvantage the agricultural and education sectors and health provision. Thirty per cent of the PA budget is committed to its security forces (Clarno, 2017: 105),[68] and in 2018 the Trump administration passed a measure that protected this sector from future cuts.[69] The premise that security should be exempt from swinging public sector cuts is well-established in past neoliberal practice; however, it also reflects the PA's general willingness to use public employment (the PA currently has 153,000 employees) 'as a pressure release valve' (Clarno, 2017: 105) to contain the complications associated with high unemployment.[70] This is among the various contradictions introduced by a neoliberal state-building that has produced various forms of dysfunction, including a pronounced democratic deficit and dependency (see Haddad, 2016).[71]

The PA is hardly in a position to challenge, let alone alter, existing distortions, as it is an essential component of the political status quo that has a clear vested interest in its continued existence. This is one of the main reasons its positions are effectively predetermined by the preferences of international actors, such as the EU. In this and other respects, it clearly recalls and resembles Gramsci's 'contradictory consciousness' that 'does not permit of any action, any decision or any choice, [producing] a condition of moral and political passivity' (1971: 641).[72] On this basis, we can presume that it will have a limited ability to respond to the economic turmoil created by the pandemic, which has caused extreme economic stress that has driven Palestinians to commit suicide.[73]

Any discussion of the Palestinian reaction to the pandemic must therefore first acknowledge and engage these different colonial dimensions. Long-standing Zionist policies converge on a simple priority, namely attaining the largest amount of Palestinian land at the 'cost' of the smallest Palestinian population. Over time, Israel's maximalist demands (recognition of West Bank settlements as part of Israel, wholesale annexation of large swathes of the West Bank and recognition of Jerusalem as the capital of Israel) have been adopted as US policy. The United States had previously, in common with the British administration, at least made an effort to maintain the appearance of even-handedness. The Trump administration makes no similar concessions.

Although economic development and modernization have historically been important parts of colonization, the extent to which the Trump administration has been willing to incorporate them into its promotion of 'peace' is entirely unprecedented. The US 'Peace to Prosperity Plan' therefore ostensibly focuses on improving the Palestinian 'quality of life' while ignoring political rights (Peace to Prosperity, 2020: 6).[74] It also emphasizes the importance of 'security criteria' established by Israel and seeks to induce the PA to (re)commit to security coordination. It is a privileged priority for all parties between August and December 2021, a time of increased settler violence, when the eviction of Sheikh Jarrah residents was threatened and a war in Gaza had recently concluded. Benny Gantz, Israel's defence minister, met with Abbas to discuss security coordination and economic issues. In the following meeting in December, Gantz promised to legalize the status of 10, 000 Palestinians who needed Israel to approve reunification documentations.[75] This was followed by a July 2022 meeting between the two that sought to offset the danger of 'instability'.[76]

US–Israel economic incentives also sought to divide Islamic Jihad and Hamas in the Strip in May 2022. One of the main reasons why Hamas stood by in the recent conflict was because it sought Israel's approval for Gazan work permits. Israel has fully grasped the political utility of economic enticements. For example, it has offered the PA Ramon Airport,[77] which is in Eilat. It opened in January 2019 but has not been operating. Palestinians see this as part of an established pattern. One Palestinian official explains that 'Israel failed to turn the Ramon Airport into an international terminal. Now the Israelis are offering us something that didn't work for them. This reminds me of the coronavirus vaccines which Israel offered us because the expiration dates were nearing'.[78]

This of course ignores the fact that the 'conflict' is political and will only be resolved on this basis. Other aid providers similarly ignore this, along with the wider colonial context. In August 2022, the EU sent €20 million to the PA to cover the cost of vaccination and an economic crisis that had escalated during the pandemic. In doing so, it did not, however, refer to the wider colonial context. Maria Velasco, the deputy EU representative, explains:

> We have been at the forefront of the international efforts to curb the pandemic by ensuring access to vaccines across the globe, including here in Palestine. The EU contributed, in this respect, both by contributing to the global initiative 'COVAX' which Palestine benefited from, and with the EUR 20 million support to the Palestinian COVID-19 vaccination campaign, as direct financial support provided

to the Palestinian Authority. With this payment, the EU reaffirms its commitment to support the building of accountable institutions ready for an independent, democratic and viable future Palestinian state.[79]

However, aid was quite clearly provided with the aim of pressurizing the PA to comply with Israeli requests. This was shown when the Institute for Monitoring Peace and Cultural Tolerance in School Education (IMPACT-se), an Israeli non-profit organization that examines school curriculums with the aim of tackling radicalism, published a 2021 report that accused Palestinians of inciting violence and establishing a curriculum that tolerated and even promoted anti-Semitism.[80] This report also criticized an EU-funded report that claimed the Palestinian curriculum met UNESCO standards.[81] In referring to this report, the EU considered cutting funding for Palestinian education.[82]

These abstract debates float above a colonial reality that persists, including in Israel, where, astonishingly, there are still no Arabic language health guidelines or information on the pandemic.[83] Some Palestinian citizens of the country claim the disinterest and inaction of the Israeli authorities, including in high levels of crime and violence, is deliberate and is intended to force them to 'leave the country of their own will'.[84] Heneida Ghanem, an activist and director of the MADAR Center, an independent research centre that specializes in Israeli affairs, traces the contemporary situation of Arabs in Israel to a Jewish supremacy that was not even qualified by the granting of Palestinian citizenship.[85] On 18 May 2021, they supported a general strike against Israeli colonialism.[86] Meanwhile, around 30,000 Palestinian Bedouins (see Nasasra, 2017),[87] who are citizens of Israel, are protesting against their proposed expulsion from land that the Jewish National Fund[88] is proposing to re-forest.[89]

In reflecting on these and other developments, it is almost impossible to avoid colonial analogies, precedents and parallels. For example, in reflecting on the pandemic, I immediately recalled Fanon's observation that '[i]n the colonial situation, therefore, it is impossible to create the physical and psychological conditions for the learning of hygiene or for the assimilation of concepts concerning epidemic diseases' (1994: 139).[90] And it should be added that '[s]ettler colonialism also has direct psychological implications as a distinct form of historical trauma characterized by intentional, ongoing assaults on collective well-being, identity, and survival' (Hammoudeh et al., 2020: 86).[91] In the Palestinian context at least, colonialism can be added to Judith Butler's list of contemporary vices ('radical inequality, nationalism and capitalist exploitation') that have found 'ways to reproduce and strengthen themselves within the pandemic zones'.[92]

These 'vices' are quite clearly interrelated. Researchers who considered pandemic developments in Middle Eastern countries (including Algeria, Iraq, Lebanon, Morocco, Sudan and Tunisia) concluded that economic crisis and inequalities enabled the virus to spread. They accordingly assert '[the pandemic is] not simply a public health crisis in and of itself' (Hanieh and Ziadeh, 2022: 22).[93] We also see this when we refer to other colonial contexts. The Red Nation (a coalition that includes native and non-native activists) observes:

> Native people are under constant assault by a capitalist-colonial logic that seeks the erasure of non-capitalist ways of life. Colonial economies interrupt cooperation and association and force people instead into hierarchical relations with agents of colonial authority who function as a permanent occupying force on Native lands.[94]

In this book, I propose that Israel's settler colonial project should be viewed as a form of 'necropolitics' that is pushing Palestinians towards 'bare life' (Agamben, 1998: 81–6).[95] Mbembe further elaborates that this 'politics' subjugates life 'to the power of death' and creates 'death-worlds'. In his words, 'late-modern colonial occupation is a concatenation of multiple powers: disciplinary, biopolitical, and necropolitical' (Mbembe, 2003: 29)[96] that render its victims as the 'living dead' (Mbembe, 2003: 40).[97]

The colonial character of the conflict is further reiterated when Israelis regurgitate the colonial fiction of *terra nullius*. Consider the example of Danny Danon, the country's former ambassador to the

UN: 'You cannot annex something that belongs to you. When you annex something you do it from a foreign territory. I do not know from whom we are annexing it.'[98] Similarly, also refer to Netanyahu's promise to advance the annexation plan[99] that was based on the 'Peace to Prosperity Plan'[100] that the United States released in January 2020. In accordance with the established colonial style, Kushner, Trump's Middle East advisor, worked on the plan for two years in total secrecy, in close cooperation with Israeli leaders but did not deign to consult Palestinians. Before releasing it, the United States took unilateral steps that favoured Israel, including moving the US Embassy to Jerusalem and cutting UNRWA funding in 2018.[101]

More recently, the East Jerusalem neighbourhood of Sheikh Jarrah, where Israel is trying to use a court order to evict Palestinians from their homes,[102] has emerged as a flashpoint in colonial conflict. In mid-April 2021, clashes erupted when Israel tried to prevent Palestinians from sitting on steps outside the Damascus Gate. In the following month, the situation further escalated and 300 Palestinians were injured after clashes between Israeli police and Palestinians. Israel's attacks on the Gaza Strip, which had catastrophic consequences for Gazans,[103] then followed. My own friends and family were affected by the 'fall-out' from the May events,[104] including by settler attacks later in the year.[105]

From the outset, I wanted this to be a book about the colonial dimensions and aspects of the pandemic. I also instead viewed it as a way of 'tapping into' and exploring related concerns, such as the state of the Palestinian health system under occupation, the past history of health provision in the territories and the politics of health.

In this book, I will discuss how 'facts on the ground', and associated predicaments, have confronted Palestinians in the pandemic. In particular, I will seek to demonstrate how colonial activities and Israeli policies have impacted the ability of Palestinians to fight the virus. I will draw on theories of settler colonialism to analyse the policies that seek to control Palestinian land and population (Wolfe, 1999: 1, 2006: 388–9; Veracini 2010: 33,101, 2011: 1 and Mamdani 2015: 610).[106] In doing so, I will demonstrate how checkpoints, bypass roads, settlement construction and the Apartheid Wall implement and reproduce a fragmentary 'logic of elimination' that can be traced back to Israel's establishment.[107]

I would like to more closely examine how colonizing policies pursued under the pretext of neoliberal 'reform' have influenced the Palestinian response to the pandemic. In doing so, I would like to consider how the mindsets and predispositions created by the colonial context of the West Bank and Gaza have left Palestinians more exposed to the virus. By, for example, developing and applying the concept of 'necropolitics', I will consider the emergence of 'death-worlds' that render Palestinians as the 'living dead'. My case studies will demonstrate how colonial policies that have created 'a permanent condition of "being in pain"' (Mbembe, 2003: 39)[108] have made Palestinians less concerned about the threats and hazards associated with the pandemic.

I refer to case studies and interviews. Palestinian interviewees, including healthcare professionals and activists, provide an extensive insight into living under colonial policies and the pandemic. By enabling Palestinian voices, I will provide critical insight into the impact of colonial policies on ongoing Palestinian efforts to survive and confront the pandemic.

My positionality

In engaging and relaying these collective experiences, my status as a Palestinian who has lived under settler colonialism is important because this reassures interviewees that I understand their positions and specifically their position in relation to dominant knowledge (Abu Saad, 2008: 1907; Smith, 2012).[109] In this regard, my focus on 'documenting real practical experiences'[110] helped to reassure them. I also felt that interviewees clearly understood that the purpose of my research is to resist colonization (Smith, 2012: 10, 29).

At the start of the interviews, most interviewees asked me if I lived in Palestine and was familiar with the situation. Some of the interviewees did not explicitly refer to certain events or parties but instead used codes that are only known to Palestinians. When my interviews with Gazans were interrupted, there was no need for them to explain if it was due to a power cut or fighting as they knew I already understood, as they implicitly acknowledged when they used phrases such as 'you know' or included me in their references to Palestinians.

However, in contrast to my interviewees, I did not make this assumption and indeed regarded myself as something of an 'outsider' (I have not lived in the West Bank since 2011) when listening to them describe key events and developments. However, some of my interviewees perhaps implicitly acknowledged this when they referred to how things had changed in the territories or asked me when I last visited the Strip (in 1999).

My actual location is somewhere between the two points, as I regard myself as an activist who challenges power and domination. I am, for example, a member of the Intellectual Committee of Palestine Forum,[111] which brings together Palestinian academics, arts and intellectuals from the oPt, historical Palestine and other countries. I publish in the Arabic language and do not come with a 'tourist agenda', and nor do I adjust my research to reflect academic fashions (Tamari, 1995).[112] I anticipate that my positionality will enable me to reveal 'the truth that was prioritized, in view of the ongoing Palestinian national struggle for liberation' (Al-Hardan, 2014: 66).[113]

Over time, I built a rapport with my interviewees – as the situation in the Strip escalated,[114] we stayed in touch via social media and I even consoled them when they lost loved ones. Over the course of our conversations, interviewees came to see that my research 'includes the moment of the production of academic truths, the making of texts, and the representation of Palestinian lives' (Al-Hardan, 2014: 67).[115] This was clearly understood and appreciated by my interviewees, many of whom stayed in touch and continued to pass me information, even after the interviews finished.

The value of this type of research is clearly recognized by the Māori scholar Linda Tuhiwai Smith:

Engaging in a discussion about research as an indigenous issue has been about finding a voice, or a way of voicing concerns, fears, desires, aspirations, needs and questions as they relate to research. When indigenous people become the researchers and not merely the researched, the activity of research is transformed. Questions are framed differently, priorities are ranked differently, problems are defined differently, people participate on different terms. (Smith, 2012: 193)

Through my engagement with the work of Smith and other critical observers of settler colonialism, I came to appreciate the truth of Abu Saad's claim: '[T]he dominant group tended to know only its own understanding of reality and social relations because it had ignored, rejected, and silenced the differing perspectives of those over whom it had power.' (2008: 1906). And I similarly came to comprehend his assertion that 'how skewed the discourse can become when neutrality is determined from the perspective of the dominant standpoint alone, in absence of an analysis of the power relations it is used to describe or disguise' (2008: 1914).

My work therefore seeks to challenge colonial ideology and epistemologies, and strives to establish the meaning of decolonization for the colonized. I view a decolonizing methodology as part of the native's struggle to achieve justice. Adherence to Western methodologies in research has resulted in native narratives being sacrificed to objectivity and the oversight of disparities and oppression. Palestinian researchers also emphasize the role of history in helping to challenge colonial actions, views and claims. Smith acknowledges this when she asserts: '[Natives] have a different epistemological tradition which frames the way we see the world, the way we organize ourselves in it, the questions we ask and the solutions we seek' (2012: 187–8).[116] However, external observers frequently resist the significance and implications of historical context. The ahistorical Oslo Accords are one example. And *The Peace to Prosperity Plan* actually asserts this oversight as a precondition for the resolution of the 'conflict'. It asserts that '[r]eciting past narratives about the conflict is unproductive. In order to resolve this conflict, the solution must be forward-looking and dedicated to the improvement of security and quality of life, while being respectful of the historic and religious significance of the region to its peoples' (6).[117]

In tracing a line that runs from the Balfour Declaration (which notoriously referred to Palestinians as 'non-Jewish' populations of Palestine) to the Oslo Accords,[118] we can identify how colonial mechanisms of control were, in a transition from colonialism to neocolonialism, gradually refined and developed. Categorization, an unbridled faith in the efficacy of military force and Jewish supremacy were essential accompaniments.

The Oslo Accords have contributed to the splintering of the Palestinian national movement and to the emergence of five distinct Palestinian constituencies (Palestinian residents in Israel, Gaza, Jerusalem, the West Bank and in exile) who are confronted by very different political challenges. In the post-Oslo years, the divides between the West Bank and Jerusalem have been formalized, as Israel's de facto annexation of territories beyond the 'separation wall' confirms.

The Israeli authorities had long recognized that Palestinians under occupation were more likely to compromise and therefore invested every effort, including ensuring that divisions and subdivisions were visually embodied on car number plates and ID cards. In displaying a similar attention to detail, the Israeli authorities also tried to cultivate and exploit emerging divides within the Palestinian national movement – the indirect support given to Hamas shortly after its establishment was just one example of this. Israel has always sought to drive a wedge between Palestinians in the oPt and those in exile, and it has done so with the aim of undermining the PLO's claim to represent all Palestinians. This imperative also guided Begin's actions (as shown by the autonomy plan) at the Camp David negotiations in 1978. However, as the past history of the peace process clearly illustrates any concession will ultimately elicit a demand for further concessions, up until the point where there is nothing more to give.

The stubborn refusal to acknowledge the region's past history is entirely understandable given the role of imperial power/s in crafting the Sykes–Picot Agreement, the Balfour Declaration and the Mandate. Like its historical predecessors, the plan's appeal to even-handedness is belied by an embedded bias. Like them, it originates in a belief that the colonizer has an unquestionable right to impose terms on the native and present them as holy writ.[119] From the outset, Zionism was defined by its close convergence with imperialism, to the point where they effectively became inseparable. Both converged on a shared desire to frustrate Palestinian national aspirations, and this became increasingly obvious as the British Mandate developed.

This historical oversight is also reproduced in a stubborn and persistent refusal to acknowledge Palestinians as equals. In this regard, it is instructive to note how the neoliberal Accords effectively co-opted Palestinian political parties, leaving them with no popular base or influence. This was particularly important because these parties had previously filled gaps in Israeli service provision (Naser-Najjab, 2020).[120]

And it is further reiterated by a rejection of the very premise of decolonized research and research perspectives. For example, the faith that the Peace Prosperity Plan invests in projects that seek to 'bring the people closer together through dialogue' (Peace to Prosperity, 2020: 35)[121] deliberately overlooks continued Palestinian objections to the very premise of dialogue-based initiatives, which are very much rooted in (negative) past experience.[122]

Book overview

I use four case studies – of the Gaza Strip, Hebron, Kuft 'Aqab and Jalazone refugee camp – to identify how the pandemic has impacted Palestinians. In referring to these and other contexts, I show that Israel is, in the manner of demagogues and political opportunists the world over, seeking to exploit the pandemic for its own purposes.

In the first chapter, I outline the historical and contemporary dimensions of colonialism in Palestine. In doing so, I reiterate and underline the contemporary significance of colonialism. For example, in referring to the PA's role in contemporary political arrangements, I seek to demonstrate how its actions (and just as often, inactions) are only intelligible when considered in relation to neoliberal reforms introduced after the Oslo Accords. In adapting and applying the notion of a 'logic of elimination', the chapter demonstrates how Israeli oversight of Palestinian existence is both willed and worked towards.

In the second chapter, I look at the pandemic's impact on the Gaza Strip by specifically referring to internal Palestinian divisions and the continued Israeli blockade. Successive wars in the Strip were, and continue to be, manipulated by external actors for their own purposes – Iran continues to support Hamas and Islamic Jihad, and Israel, the United States and the PA continue to pressurize Hamas. The impact of the recent four wars is still apparent on basic education, health and housing services, and two-thirds of Gazans have no food security. Medical and health workers have been killed, and hospitals, ambulances and primary healthcare centres have been destroyed. Meanwhile, the continued blockade makes it impossible to restore the health system to even a basic level of functionality.

The majority of Gazans are refugees and rely on UNRWA services, although cuts and neoliberal reforms have made it increasingly difficult for the agency to operate, let alone meet needs and demands. The Strip's refugee camps also provide perfect incubating environments for the virus.

The third chapter addresses Hebron, the largest governorate in the West Bank. The Hebron Protocol divided the city into H1 (PA administration) and H2 (Israeli control), which includes the South Hebron Hills, which include the Masafer Yatta area, where the 4,000 (mainly farmers and shepherds) residents of 30 villages live with the continual threat of transfer. The Israeli army is permanently stationed in H2, where, among other activities, it closes streets and sets up checkpoints and installs metal gates. Colonial activities that include demolitions, settlement plans and violent settler attacks persist, and efforts to contain the virus are obstructed by the army's deliberate destruction of Palestinian infrastructure, including facilities essential for water, sanitation and hygiene purposes.

Chapter 4 engages Kufr 'Aqab neighbourhood, which is part of Jerusalem municipality but which is 'beyond the wall'. Here there are no municipal services, and the PA is forbidden from operating here. After the Second *Intifada*, the construction of the Apartheid Wall cut the neighbourhood, which is on the 'frontline' of Israel's Judaization of Jerusalem, and is cut off from the rest of the city. Like villagers in Khan Al-Ahmar, a village near Jerusalem, the residents live with the continual threat of eviction and displacement (B'Tselem, 2018).[123] Kufr 'Aqab and other areas 'beyond the wall' are affected by poor infrastructure and a security gap, and although the PA is not permitted to operate here, the Israeli police refuse to intervene. Many residents have Jerusalem IDs but their partners have West Bank IDs, which is a further complicating factor.

The final chapter examines how the pandemic has affected Jalazone refugee camp, which was established in 1949. The camp's 10,000 inhabitants are crammed into a space of just 0.253 sq km and are afflicted by a range of health issues as a result of overcrowding, poor ventilation, the lack of a sewage system and no proper sanitary facilities. In these conditions, it is almost impossible for inhabitants to follow World Health Organization (WHO) guidelines, including on social distancing.

These case studies will provide insight into how the colonial situation, including land fragmentation and categorization, has impacted Palestinians in their everyday lives. Throughout, I continually stress and reiterate that aspects of the colonial situation, including fragmentation, should not be misunderstood as a consequence but rather as a desired action that is continually pursued and promoted by the colonial power in pursuit of broader colonial aims and objectives. In response, I ground my research in resistance and the reimagining of justice, and thereby align myself with Sabbagh-Khoury's call for forms of 'Palestinian resistance and survival' that will 'disrup[t] this structure and shap[e] its transformation' (2021: 18).[124]

Theoretical and historical background

Introduction: Theorizing colonial power

Israel made no great effort to give the impression it cared about the oPt's inhabitants. Its attitude was quite clearly some distance removed from the more 'benign' colonial predecessors that Fanon related ('colonialism pretends to consider them, recognizing with ostentatious humility that the territory is suffering from serious underdevelopment which necessitates a great economic and social effort') (1963: 208). In reality, Israel's colonial rule was 'always accompanied by an almost mechanical sense of detachment and mistrust of even the things that are most positive and most profitable to the population' (1994: 139).[1] Moshe Dayan's 'enlightened occupation' was therefore a self-serving fraud (Pappé, 2017: Chapter 7; also see Weizman, 2007: 95).[2] Even when he first introduced the concept, he knew this full well, as he could hardly be ignorant of the fact that colonialism is only ever imposed on a population. Here, I recall Trouillot's observation that 'any system of domination [has] the tendency to proclaim its own normalcy. To acknowledge resistance as a mass phenomenon is to acknowledge the possibility that something is wrong with the system' (2015: 84).[3]

The territories bear a deep colonial imprint and this attests to the fact that, at almost all points, the Zionist project was enabled and facilitated by imperialism (Derek, 2004: 79; Hilal, 1976 and Sayegh, 2012). Izzat Tanous recalls that Arthur Balfour refused to meet Arab delegates when they tried to arrange a meeting with him in Geneva in September 1921. He is on record as replying: '[I]f the Palestinian delegates want to see me concerning Palestine, let them go meet Dr Haim Weizmann'

(1982: 104). The PLO reiterated this imperial legacy in 1968 when it referred to Zionism as the product of an 'imperialist invasion' (Muslih, 1990: 9). Fayez Sayegh, a former member of the executive committee of the Palestine Liberation Organization (PLO), further clarifies that 'the political embodiment of Zionist colonialism (namely, the Zionist settler-state of Israel) is characterized chiefly by three features: (1) its racial complexion and racist conduct pattern; (2) its addiction to violence; and (3) its expansionist stance' (1965: 21).[4]

Israel's contemporary policies also firmly reiterate its settler colonial credentials (Wolfe, 1999: 1; also see Wolfe, 2006: 388–9; Veracini, 2010: 33 and101, 2011: 1 and Mamdani, 2015: 610). Transfer and elimination continue in all parts of historical Palestine, including the Galilee and Negev (see Nasasra et al., 2015; Rouhana and Sabbagh-Khoury, 2015).

A recent Amnesty International report, published on 1 February 2022, describes Israel as an apartheid state that 'treat[s] Palestinians as an inferior racial group' and adds that 'Israeli authorities enact multiple measures to deliberately deny Palestinians their basic rights and freedoms, including draconian movement restrictions in the OPT, chronic discriminatory underinvestment in Palestinian communities in Israel, and the denial of refugees' right to return'.[5]

In sketching the links between historical and contemporary colonialism, we are forced to acknowledge both essential continuities and key developments and divergences. And here it should be acknowledged that colonialism does not exclusively rely on direct physical force or coercion, as Wolfe reiterates when observing that the settler colonial 'logic of elimination' is 'not invariably genocidal' (2006: 387). And he adds the native can be eliminated in various ways by a settler colonial power that seeks to replace the native and 'stay' (Wolfe, 2006: 388).[6]

But what are these colonial features?

First, inverting reality by cultivating a bogus moral authority. Here, consider Mourid Barghouti's analysis of Rabin's speech after he signed the 1993 Oslo Accords:

It is easy to blur the truth with a simple linguistic trick: start your story from 'Secondly.' Yes, this is what Rabin did. He simply neglected to speak of what happened first. Start your story with 'Secondly,' and the world will be turned upside-down. Start your story with 'Secondly,' and the arrows of the Red Indians are the original criminals and the guns of the white men are entirely the victim. It is enough to start with 'Secondly,' for the anger of the black man against the white to be barbarous. Start with 'Secondly,' and Gandhi becomes responsible for the tragedies of the British. (2004:178/Ra'aytu Ramallah (I saw Ramallah) 195)

At this time, it was commonplace for international observers to celebrate the Accords as the achievement of an international diplomacy that had enticed the Palestinian leadership to adopt suitably 'moderate' positions. This implicitly presupposed the Palestinian leadership, and more precisely their alleged rejectionism, was the main obstacle to peace, an understanding at odds with the established historical record. The associated premise that this 'achievement' enabled the 'international community' to engage with the 'conflict' also overlooked the fact the 'conflict' was in fact internationalized from the early twentieth century onwards.[7] This inattention to basic historical facts reflects the fact that, as Said (2001) notes,[8] Zionists 'had already won the political battle for Palestine in the international world in which ideas, representation, rhetoric and images were at issue'.[9]

In referring to the standard westernized historiography, external observers could easily be forgiven for believing that the conflict began in 1967 and that Palestinian state-building within the parameters of the two-state solution is the only issue that remains to be resolved. Similarly, it is insufficiently acknowledged that the Zionist 'concession' of partition was only accepted on a provisional basis. At the time, the UN similarly obligingly overlooked this. Khalidi observes:

In retrospect, and in the light of half a century of contemplation, what is most striking about the Zionist version of the background, nature, circumstances, and aftermath of the 1947 partition resolution is the extent to which it has become the paradigm or lens through which the entire history of the Palestine problem and the Zionist-Arab conflict prior and subsequent to the resolution itself is viewed and judged. (1997: 5)

Pappé shows how 'transfer', a euphemism for ethnic cleansing, later emerged as a key component of the Zionist project after the UN passed its partition resolution (2006: Chapter 4); Masalha (1992); and Piterberg (2008). He also observes that partition was in any case impossible, as the promises made to Jews and Palestinians could not both be kept. This was confirmed by the Peel Commission:

In any scheme of dividing Palestine the primary difficulty lies in the fact that no line can be drawn which would separate all the Arabs from all the Jews. Both under cantonisation and under partition a minority of each race remains in an area controlled by a majority of the other.' (Peel Commission, 1937: Chapter XXI, p3 79). [And recommended] [i]f partition is to be effective in promoting a final settlement it must mean more than drawing a frontier and establishing two States. Sooner or later there should be a transfer of land and, as far as possible, an exchange of population. (Peel Commission, 1937: Chapter XXII, p. 389)

Given this stubborn and unyielding reality, it is no surprise that Zionists went to great lengths to conceal the contents and implications of their designs – for example, in the period between the Basel Program of 1897 and the Biltmore Program of 1942, they referred to 'home' rather than 'state' (Sayegh, 1965: 3). Fayez Sayegh, in referring to the example of Palestine, reminds us that '[w]hile the instruments of colonisation were being laboriously created, diplomatic efforts were also being exerted to produce *political conditions* that would permit, facilitate, and protect large-scale colonisation' (1965: 6).[10]

Second, land fragmentation. As already noted (see Introduction), this is not an inadvertent outcome but is instead actively desired and worked towards by the colonial power (Rishmawi, 1986; Roy, 2004).[11] It includes the 'thinning out' of the Palestinian population in the oPt that is exemplified by Israel invoking a spurious 'security' pretext to destroy areas that 'border' military zones.[12] Israel's control and surveillance mechanisms facilitate land expropriation (Weizman, 2007; Halper, 2015).[13] And a surveillance system subjects 'physical existence and spaces' to 'constant scrutiny, which provokes ongoing insecurity and anxiety' (Badarin, 2015: 234).[14] Meanwhile, Israel invokes spurious security pretexts to 'justify' the construction of checkpoints, walls and other blockades that restrict Palestinian movement. Controls expose Palestinian to the possibility of separation from the land or even eviction (Weizman, 2007; Badarin, 2015; Halper, 2015).[15]

In the 1990s, Israel used settlements and bypass roads to subdivide Palestinian communities (Roy, 2004;[16] Hilal, 2015),[17] resulting in 'Bantust-anization' (Farsakh, 2008:238)[18] and restricted economic development (2000: 54).[19] The resulting control and surveillance system that sought to restrict Palestinian movement and development (Weizman, 2007; Halper, 2015)[20] attested to the structural character of colonialism.[21]

Peace Now has estimated that in 2013 alone, Israeli settlement construction increased by 123 per cent.[22] It also asserted that the Israeli government approved the construction of new settlements that 'would enable continuous expansion of all settlements, without any limitations'.[23] Eyal Weizman acknowledges this reality when he speaks of 'shifting, fragmented and elastic territories' (2007: 4)[24] and 'multiplying archipelagos of externally alienated and internally homogenous ethno-national enclaves [that live] under a blanket of aerial Israeli surveillance' (2007: 7; also see Halper, 2015).

Fragmentation was a deliberate tactic that, in the words of Hilal, 'rendered Palestinian communities – inside historic Palestine and outside – very vulnerable, and made collective action against collective colonial repression more difficult' (2015: 1).[25] It also undermined efforts to initiate and sustain collective action (Hilal, 2015: 1),[26] restricted Palestinian movement, divided communities and inserted Palestinians into residence-based categories. Land confiscations and settlement expansion also inflicted ongoing hardships on Palestinians.

The Apartheid Wall further fragmented land and population and imposed more movement restrictions on Palestinians. After the

Al-Aqsa Intifada, the fragmentation of Palestinian land and population accelerated, as Palestinians were increasingly unable to access essential needs, such as water.[27] Movement restrictions also resulted in the emergence of enclaves (Farsakh, 2008: 238;[28] Roy, 1995: 117).[29] And the Accords effectively imposed an unaccountable and ineffective leadership on the oPt, in a manner very much consistent with colonial precedents – Alfred, in referring to the example of Canada, therefore observes that 'the state has nothing to fear from Native leaders. [E]ven if they succeed in achieving the goal of self-government, the basic power structure remains intact' (1999: 71).[30] He subsequently presents peace agreements as a settler colonial tactic intended to control and ultimately replace natives (2010: 33). [31]

The Accords therefore effectively denied the essential truth that 'a better colonial order is better but it is not a noncolonial one' (Veracini 2011: 5).[32] Far from enabling separation, ensuing arrangements actually strengthened Israel's control over the territories (Veracini, 2010: 45).[33] When thousands of military orders control almost all aspects of everyday life (JMCC, 1993),[34] 'development' actually increases the oPt's dependence on Israel (Rishmawi, 1986; Tamari, 1988).[35]

Third, the establishment of a compliant and weak local leadership that implements a 'divide and rule' strategy. Here it is instructive to note that it was Oslo II that inserted Palestinians in different categories and, in so doing, subjected them to various different administrative rules (see Roy, 2004 and Hilal, 2015).[36] The PA's extensive patron–client arrangements (around 40 per cent of the PA budget is spent on salaries) co-opt a substantial part of this Palestinian population (Al-Shu'aibi, 2012; Al-Masri, 2016), as the PA recognized when it responded to persistent Fatah–Hamas tensions by cutting the salaries of Hamas government employees in the Gaza Strip (Roy 2017; Tibon 2018).

The establishment of the PA reflected and upheld the privileging of security as a political priority. The peace process and negotiations mainly focused on security issues, and the United States and other international donors made it clear the PA would only continue to receive funding if Israel's security demands and conditions were met (Haddad, 2016). In referring to the Wye River Memorandum, Aruri observes that '[t]he section on security consumes about 60 percent of the memorandum, while the rest [addresses] further redeployment (itself linked to security needs) and unresolved interim issues' (1999: 18).

From the start of the Oslo negotiations, Israel redefined the meaning of security and expected Palestinian to unquestioningly accept this. As Memmi observes, 'The crushing of the colonized is included among the colonizer's values. As soon as the colonized adopts those values, he similarly adopts his own condemnation.'[37] This perpetuates and sustains the colonial structure.[38]

In the secret negotiations that established the Oslo Accords, Uri Savir cautioned against any proposed rapprochement between Fatah and Hamas (2005: 250)[39] and encouraged Arafat to 'take concrete steps against terrorist elements on the ground' (2005: 250).[40] Hershfield, the Israeli academic who initiated the secret negotiations, told Ahmad Qurei', the chief Palestinian negotiator: 'Terrorism is escalating steadily, not only from Hamas, but other groups from the PLO, we need an effective coordination to control violence' (Qurei', 2005: 101).[41] In the following years, Israel also tried to define, and ultimately frustrate, any agreement between Hamas and Fatah.[42] Savir said:

> Some of our officers were critical of Arafat because his people were placing far too much emphasis on their talks with Hamas leadership, which were taking place in Sudan with our approval. They said that it was not sufficient for Arafat to attempt to convince his ideological opponents to become a political nonviolent movement but that he should at the same time take concrete steps against terrorist elements on the ground. (1998: 250)[43]

Qurei objected that the Israelis sought to humiliate Palestinians 'by changing the word humiliation for security'.[44] However, Arafat ultimately indicated his agreement in a 1993 letter to Rabin, which stated 'the PLO renounces the use of terrorism and other acts of violence and will assume responsibility over all PLO elements and personnel in order to assure their compliance, prevent violations and discipline violators'.[45]

After the collapse of the Camp David negotiations,[46] the outbreak of the Second *Intifada* and the 11 September 2001 terrorist attacks, Israel intensified its own 'counter-terrorism' efforts.[47] Its targeting and assassination of Hamas leaders[48] threatened to undermine its working understanding with the PA by further undermining Hamas–PA relations (Roy, 2011: Chapter 7).[49] Israel therefore has to strike a delicate balance when applying its own repressive measures, lest this undermine or otherwise act to the detriment of the PA.

After the Second *Intifada*, Israel used land fragmentation and the cultivation of division to create different categories of Palestinians (Hilal, 2015).[50] This was accompanied by a state-building project that effectively regarded the occupation and its colonial dynamics as an inconvenient fact that could be worked around. This understanding was not questioned or challenged, and was indeed reproduced, by a Palestinian elite class that had, in the words of Fanon, willingly consented to 'every means to put them to sleep'. (p. 169)[51] (see also Hilal, 2010).[52]

Frantz Fanon clearly anticipated this and other similar developments when, in criticizing an earlier generation of nationalist political parties, he observed that 'the will to break colonialism is linked with another quite different will: that of coming to friendly agreement with it' (1963: 124).[53] And in Palestine, this is quite clearly indicated by the fact that peace-building and neoliberal state-building structures and processes (Khalidi and Sobhi, 2011: 15) are intended to 'coexis[t] with the operative colonial structure instead of bringing it to a close' (Badarin, 2015: 159).[54]

In June 1967, and as part of the settler colonialist state's attempt to reconcile the Israeli wish to remain demographically a Jewish state while at the same time expand geographically without losing the pretence of being a democratic state in the post-1967 reality' (Pappé, 2013: 341).[55]

The associated emergence and development of the PA marginalized the PLO, and this feature became particularly pronounced after Mahmoud Abbas simultaneously led Fatah, the PA and the PLO. After the failure of the Camp David negotiations in 2000 and the eruption of the *Al-Aqsa Intifada* in September of the same year, donors put forward a reform plan with the aim of undermining Yasser Arafat. When he died on 11 November 2004, the PA was highly dependent on external donors and Palestinian politics was deeply divided, making it difficult for political parties to pursue independent agendas (Hammami 1995). In 2005, the PA also accepted Israel's request that the definition of 'terrorism' should be expanded to include any form of Palestinian resistance (Swisher, 2011).

In June 2007, Hamas seized the Gaza Strip (Tartir, 2015)[56] before international donors introduced a security-focused reform agenda later in the same year (Clarno, 2017: 165).[57] In the period 2007–10, the United States allocated more than $392 million (USD) to counter-terrorism operations. The United States changed its funding criteria and several other donors made it clear that funding would be withheld from those who employed supporters or members of Hamas. Humanitarian and development organizations were now increasingly obliged to work within the parameters set by security coordination (Fast, 2006).[58]

Information provided by the Palestinian security forces enabled Israel to target, arrest and kill Palestinian activists. In 2017, for example, the activist Basel Al-Araj was arrested by PA forces and was assassinated by Israeli troops later in the same year (Abdalla, 2017).[59]

The *Palestine Papers* that were released in 2011 revealed that Israel asked the PA minister of the interior to kill a Fatah member of the *Al-Aqsa* Martyrs' Brigade (Swisher, 2011: 53).[60]

Financial arrangements and enticements help to solidify and perpetuate these political arrangements, as they prevent the PA from tackling colonization or trying to hold Israel to account, even if it wanted to. For example, when the PA joined the International Criminal Court (ICC) in 2015, the Israeli government retaliated by withholding Palestinian tax revenues. The PA in turn threatened to halt security coordination. John Kerry, the US Secretary of State, tried to intervene in the escalating dispute. He observed that security coordination was at risk of being suspended, and this could cause a 'crisis' that could impact the security of 'both Palestinians and Israelis' (Beaumont, 2015).[61] The combination of 'disciplinary' or 'regulatory' political and economic restrictions has in turn inhibited the PA's efforts to tackle the virus and to address economic hardship and ongoing challenges that include isolation and vaccination arrangements.[62]

Fourth, a qualified recognition that is actually a co-option. Coulthard alludes to this when he observes that '[i]n the Canadian context, colonial relations of power are no longer reproduced primarily through overtly coercive means, but rather through the asymmetrical exchange of mediated forms of state recognition and accommodation' (2014: 15).[63] These are 'nonreciprocal forms of recognition either imposed on or granted to [the colonised] by the settler state and society' (2014: 25).[64]

Qualified recognition is, by definition, partial and incomplete, which clearly recalls Fanon's account of the 'colonized' native:

> Exploitation, tortures, raids, racism, collective liquidations. rational oppression take turns at different levels in order literally to make of the native an object in the hands of the occupying nation. This object man, without means of existing, without a raison d'etre, is broken in the very depth of his substance. The desire to live, to continue, becomes more and more indecisive, more and more phantom-like. (1967 [1964]: 35)[65]

Settler colonialism is focused on land rather than the direct exploitation of the native and is distinguished from colonialism on this basis (Wolfe, 1999: 1; Wolfe, 2006: 388–9; Veracini, 2010: 33 and101, 2011: 1 and Mamdani, 2015: 610). We can accordingly speak of '[t]erritoriality [as] settler colonialism's specific, irreducible element' (Wolfe, 2006: 388). And this is precisely why colonial occupation has been defined as

> a matter of seizing, delimiting, and asserting control over a physical geographical area and of inscribing a new set of social and spatial relations on it. This writing of new spatial relations (territorialization) made it necessary to produce boundaries and hierarchies, zones and enclaves; subvert established property arrangements; classify people into different categories; extract resources; and manufacture a large reservoir of cultural imaginaries. (Mbembe, 2003: 25–6)[66]

In the case of Palestinians, the assimilationist policies of US colonization (Dunbar-Ortiz and Gilio-Whitaker, 2016: 55)[67] were clearly not on the Zionist agenda. Its strict division of populations more clearly recalls and resembles Fanon's observation that '[t]he colonial world is a Manichean world (1963: 43) "[that is] divided into compartments"' (1963: 37)[68] (also see Makdisi, 2010; and Veracini, 2010: 22[69]).

Pappé further elaborates:

> At first the area was divided into 'Arab' and potential 'Jewish' spaces. Those areas densely populated with Palestinians became autonomous, run by local collaborators under a military rule. This regime was only replaced with a civil administration in 1981. The other areas, the 'Jewish' spaces, were colonized with Jewish settlements and military bases. (2017)[70]

The rewriting of history has accompanied this territorial reimagining and has indeed been synonymous with it. The colonizer always tries to 'falsify history, he rewrites laws, he would extinguish memories – anything to succeed in transforming his usurpation into legitimacy' (1974: 96).[71] The detachment of the *Nakba* from the peace process is just one example (Hilal, 2015: 2).[72]

It is therefore no surprise, and is indeed to be expected, that Israel has not yet acknowledged its internal colonization (Rouhana and Sabbagh-Khoury, 2015; Nasasra et al., 2015),[73] and this is clearly shown by the fact that the Israeli curriculum and textbooks deny both the *Nakba* and the Palestinian narrative of other past events (Abed Elrazik, Amin and Davis, 1978).[74] Israeli learning materials contain no mention of how dispossessed Palestinians became 'present absentees' and were subject to discriminatory laws that are still active. This effective denial or collective 'unremembering' anticipates and sustains discriminatory legislation, including the 2018 Jewish nation-state law (Adala, 2020),[75] which states that 'the Land of Israel is the historical homeland of the Jewish people' and asserts that Israeli settlements are 'a national value' (Jabareen and Bishara, 2019: 55).[76] New legal measures include the 2011 Admissions Committees Law, which establishes a legal basis for rejecting Palestinian citizen applications for housing in Israel's towns and communities if they are 'unsuited' to the community's 'social life' or the town's 'social and cultural fabric'.[77] Palestinians in the unrecognized villages of the Negev who struggle for legal recognition also continue to be subject to ongoing colonial activities (Rouhana and Sabbagh-Khoury, 2015; Nasasra et al., 2015: Nasasra, 2017)[78] and related discrimination. Badarin explains this activity is 'essentially eliminatory' (2015: 4),[79] even if it does not involve the actual physical elimination of the Palestinian population. This recalls a quote from Foucault: 'When I say "killing", I obviously do not mean simply murder as such, but also every form of indirect murder: the fact of exposing someone to death, increasing the risk of death for some people, or, quite simply, political death, expulsion, rejection, and so on' (2003a: 256).[80]

Theorizing necropolitics and biopolitics

In this book, I draw on and apply the concept of 'necropolitics' to explain how the Israeli settler colonial project is pushing Palestinians towards 'bare life' (Agamben, 1998: 81–6).[81] Agamben, in referring to a 'bare life' that 'blinds and separates', further elaborates this concept:

> We have become so accustomed to living in conditions of perennial crisis and perennial emergency that we do not seem to notice that life is being reduced to a purely biological condition in which the social and political – even the human and emotional – dimensions are lost.[82]

I will also refer to Mbembe's concept of necropolitics, which involves the 'subjugation of life to the power of death' and the creation of 'death-worlds' where populations endure destruction and death. In doing so, I will refer to a system of surveillance that has developed since Israel first introduced Palestinian ID cards (that identified holders on the basis of their place of residence) after the 1967 War (Tawol-Souri, 2011).[83]

The concept of necropolitics derives from Michel Foucault's 'biopolitics'. Foucault once spoke of Biopolitics as a tool that would make it possible to control and dominate the 'population' at all times (2003a: 244)[84] and as the enactment of 'the right to make live and to let die' (2003a: 40–1). For Foucault, health interventions did not, in a naïve fashion, simply seek to preserve 'life'. Instead, he viewed them as a way of classifying, dehumanizing, excluding and eliminating. In order to grasp this, first refer to his distinction between 'negative' ('a technology of power that drives out, excludes, banishes, marginalizes, and represses') and 'positive' ('that fashions, observes, knows, and multiplies itself on the basis of its own effects' (2003b: 48)) power.[85] In referring to 'power' in the context of health interventions, Foucault spoke of a 'biopolitics of population' that entailed the 'explosion of numerous and diverse techniques for achieving the subjugation of bodies and the control of populations' (1990: 140),[86] and held that threats would henceforth be engaged on the premise they 'represent a kind of biological danger' (1978: 138).[87]

He further elaborates that power operates in an

[E]nclosed, segmented space, observed at every point, in which the individuals are inserted in a fixed place, in which the slightest movements are supervised, in which all events are recorded, in which an uninterrupted work of writing links the centre and periphery, in which power is exercised without division, according to a continuous hierarchical figure, in which each individual is constantly located, examined and distributed among the living beings, the sick and the dead. (1991: 197)[88]

Morgensen explains that '[t]he biopolitics of settler colonialism sustain[s] the persistence of settler states, and we must interpret their activities as precisely enacting settler colonialism' (Morgensen, 2013: 71).[89] In the oPt, we can therefore identify a 'concatenation of multiple powers, disciplinary, biopolitical and necropolitical' (Mbembe, 2003: 29) that operate in both time and space (Daher-Nashif, 2021).[90] Foucault implicitly acknowledged this when, in stressing the interrelation of power and resistance, he referred to 'a multiplicity of points of resistance' that 'are present everywhere in the power network' (Foucault, 1990:

95–6).[91] Foucault spoke of a 'biopolitics of population' that entailed the 'explosion of numerous and diverse techniques for achieving the subjugation of bodies and the control of populations' (1990: 140). Threats, he suggested, would henceforth be addressed on the grounds that they 'represent a kind of biological danger' (1978: 138).[92]

This clearly recalls the way that Israel's security apparatus has 'mobilized' in response to the pandemic. The Israeli authorities have, in invoking the pandemic as a pretext, activated a counterterrorism database (created in 2002) with the aim of tracking citizens and ensuring they adhere to lockdown regulations. This is another illustration of how the pandemic provided Israel with an opportunity to enhance its scrutiny of Palestinians.

Given this, it is clearly not unreasonable to presume that Israel will use cybersurveillance to target activists and human rights organizations. The prominence of Mossad in the State's pandemic response also underlines that 'it is only natural for a national security state like Israel to see Covid-19 as a security threat just as much or more than a health threat'.[93] This understanding is also invoked in Shalhoub–Kevorkian's (2015) allusion to a 'security theology' (2015)[94] that is part of 'the processes and mechanisms that support the ability to reorder, regulate and discipline bodies and lives' (2015: 5).[95]

Ghanim (2008), however, argues that the concept of biopower does not provide full insight into colonial policies in Palestine, and instead proposes thanatopower as a better theoretical framework. It is, she notes, 'called to action at those delicate moments of passage from calculating life to calculating death, from managing life to managing death, and from the politicization of life to the politicization of death' (2008: 68).[96] In referring to the Strip's 'state of exception' that has been exacerbated since 2007, along with Israel's refusal to permit life-saving treatment to Gazans with chronic illnesses (B'Tselem, 2021),[97] she observes '[u]nder colonial occupation, the lives of subjects are expropriated. They are exposed to the continual threat of death that becomes a permanent shadow accompanying them. Death is just on hold, again and again, from moment to moment' (Ghanim, 2008: 67). This clearly captures how Palestinians effectively live under a suspended death sentence, as I will subsequently demonstrate in more detail.

Theorizing resistance

Theory should not only seek to provide insight into the precise features and dimensions of colonialism but should also, to the same extent, seek to sketch the outlines of future resistance. Palestinians historically viewed their resistance to Israeli colonialism as part of a wider anti-colonial struggle,[98] as Sayegh acknowledges in asserting that Palestinians historically viewed 'the cause of anti-colonialism and liberation [a]s one and indivisible'. (Sayegh, 1965: 51). In reiterating this, Angela Davis insists on the '[i]ntersectionality of struggle' (2016: 144)[99] and asserts that '[i]t is in collectivities that we find reservoirs of hope and optimism' (2016: 49).

For example, the indigenous leader Waziyatawin, who is from Pezihutazizi Otunwe (Yellow Medicine Village) in southwestern Minnesota, visited Palestine in 2011 as part of a 'solidarity' delegation. She later wrote that her people were inspired by Palestinian resistance. In her words, 'withstand[ing] ongoing occupation requires never losing sight of the end-goal of liberation and fiercely engaging and supporting acts of resistance' (2012: 182).[100]

Salamanca et al. add:

> Such an alignment would expand the tools available to Palestinians and their solidarity movement, and reconnect the struggle to its own history of anti-colonial internationalism. At its core, this internationalist approach asserts that the Palestinian struggle against Zionist settler colonialism can only be won when it is embedded within, and empowered by, broader struggles – all anti-imperial, all anti-racist, and all struggling to make another world possible. (2012: 5)[101]

But this in turn raises the question of what form this conjoined struggle should take. Dunbar-Ortiz, in referring to the example of the United

States, observes how indigenous communities 'survive and bear witness to this history' (2014: 7).[102] However, while natives seek to challenge colonial structures and terms (Coulthard, 2014),[103] they are ultimately cast in the (paradoxical) role of seeking to 'negotiate a relation of nondomination with a structure of domination like the colonial nation-state' (Coulthard, 2014: 159).[104] This is clearly problematic as they ultimately do not seek some sort of 'reconciliation' with colonialism but rather strive to '[c]reate a new reality' (Alfred, 2005: 19)[105] that is based on their own vision of justice (Simpson, 2011: 17).[106] The Canadian indigenous movement Idle No More stressed this when it 'called on all people to join in a peaceful revolution which honours and fulfills Indigenous sovereignty and which protects the land, the water, and the sky' (Idle No More website).[107]

While resistance on this scale is clearly a formidable undertaking, there are successful precedents. In 2020, the US Supreme Court recognized the Native American claim to half of Oklahoma's land.[108] The Sioux tribe's struggle to regain land that the United States confiscated in 1877 was also ultimately recognized by a US Supreme Court ruling that offered millions of dollars in compensation. However, the Sioux refused the compensation on the grounds 'the land was never for sale'. Dunbar-Ortiz reflects that this example 'demonstrates the relevance and significance of the land to the Sioux, not as an economic resource but as a relationship between people and place, a profound feature of the resilience of the Indigenous peoples of the Americas' (2014: 208).[109]

In his autobiography, Elias Nasrallah, a Palestinian citizen of Israel, echoes this sentiment when he recalls a conversation with his nephew over their inherited land that was taken by the Israelis. His nephew refused to accept the prospect that the inherited land could not be distributed, and said 'today our land is confiscated but no one knows what would happen later and I want my share of this land, even if it is returned back after 1000 years' (2016: 672).[110]

Genuine decolonization therefore rejects the very notion of compromise with the status quo, and this is why Fanon spoke of it as a 'program of complete disorder' (1963: 63).[111] This is also the essential meaning that Tuck & Yang aspire to when they assert that decolonization is 'unsettling because it is not a metaphor'. When the reverse happens, and 'metaphor invades decolonization, it kills the very possibility of decolonization; it recenters whiteness, it resettles theory, it extends innocence to the settler, it entertains a settler future' (2012: 3).[112] And this is precisely why 'decolonization in the settler colonial context must repatriate land and surmount the limitations of a symbolic adjustment' (2012: 7).

The Boycott, Divestment and Sanctions (BDS) movement advances demands in similar terms and does not entertain the prospect of concessions to colonial power (Qumsiyeh, 2016).[113] It has redefined Palestinian struggle and mobilized Palestinians from across historical Palestine.

Sara Roy explains:

> [BDS] has as its main component nonviolent mass mobilization around a rights-based agenda that solicits support from the international community, including Israel. This includes a renewed campaign around the refugee right of return, which has reasserted itself after years of absence during the Oslo period; a boycott and divestment movement; and a strengthened relationship between Palestinians in the occupied territories and the Palestinian citizens of Israel. (2012: 87)

Hilal also suggests change could emerge from material developments. He observes:

> [C]umulative conditions pushing for collective popular action, leading to organized popular resistance against the Israeli colonial occupation, should not be excluded, given the entrenchment of the political deadlock and the policy of collective repression and punishment, as well as the ongoing intensification of colonization and national humiliation, and an extremely right-wing Israeli government. (2015: 9)[114]

In resisting submission to this 'bare life', Palestinians have established community solidarity campaigns focused on the vulnerable. One example was the Union of Agricultural Work Committees (UAWC) that distributed food and hygiene supplies to families in the Strip.[115]

Nasr Abdel Karim, a professor of finance and economics, also suggested to the Ministry of Agriculture that agricultural engineers should encourage home gardens as a way of meeting food and economic needs at the peak of the pandemic.[116]

The pandemic also encouraged Palestinians to reimagine resistance. UAWC's 'United Against COVID-19' campaign, called on Palestinians to 'go back to the land and cultivate it.'[117] UAWC also cooperates with international alliances to generate international solidarity and support. It is a member of the La Via Campesina, an international movement that serves as 'a platform for its members worldwide to communicate and carry out joint solidarity actions, mobilizations, and campaigns in defence of land, water, seeds, and forests.'[118] During lockdown, it could only operate virtually. This is just one example of how Covid-19 has contributed to important creative innovations in Palestinian resistance to post-*Nakba* colonialism.

And in May 2021, Palestinian resistance managed to halt the eviction of Palestinians from the East Jerusalem neighbourhood of Sheikh Jarrah and settlements in Kufr 'Aqab. Social media was an important part of this mobilization – for example, the hashtag #SaveSheikhJarrah enabled Palestinians to post images and videos of brutal attacks on Palestinian civilians. As a result, many celebrities and prominent figures expressed their solidarity with protesting Palestinians.

Israel's health provision in the oPt

In the pre-Oslo period, Israel was responsible for different aspects of Palestinian health care in hospitals and clinics, including employment and supplies. It provided a very limited budget for basic services focused on primary health care and did not acknowledge an ongoing need for secondary and tertiary care. After the 1967 war, rising numbers of polio cases provided it with an incentive to provide health care, and this again confirmed Fanon's insight that the colonizer 'never gives anything away for nothing' (1963: 142). Teddy Kollek acknowledged this when he scornfully dismissed the proposition that he had served Arab communities during his tenure as mayor of Jerusalem in the period 1965–93:

> Idiocy, fairy tales! I did nothing over the last 20 years. For Jewish Jerusalem I have done things. For East Jerusalem? Nothing? Stop babbling about sidewalks, cultural centers. Nothing! Absolutely nothing! Actually, we did build the sewage system and improved the water system. And do you know why? I'm sure you think we did it for their benefit. No way! We did it because we heard about cholera cases, and the Jews feared the spread of an epidemic. (quoted in Hodgkins, 1998: 67)

In the pre-Oslo period, and especially during the First *Intifada*, Palestinians were effectively obliged to provide health care on the basis of communal solidarity. The Unified National Leadership of the Uprising (UNLU), for example, called on 'all those physicians, pharmacists, and nurses who have already given great support to our cause, to continue their tireless efforts at providing emergency relief and routine medical care to the people. (Toward a State of Independence, 1988: 101).[119]

Grassroots medical committees provided medical relief and first aid, and medical team visited villages and camps under curfew after trekking through mountains to avoid checkpoints. Medical care work included testing the water tanks to check for any deliberate contamination by the Israeli army. Medical groups worked with Makkasid Hospital and Bethlehem University to collect information about injuries caused by the Israeli army. They assessed those with life-changing injuries and established a community-based rehabilitation (CBR) programme.[120]

In the post-Oslo period, Palestinians were increasingly pressurized by external donors to partner with Israelis on medical projects and joint initiatives. For example, the PA's November 2020 decision to resume security coordination, which included transferring patients to Israel to receive treatment, was praised by the UN.[121]

Such 'encouragement', however, appeared to defy the conclusions of researchers that this and other similar initiatives strengthened Israel's (colonial) control over the West Bank.[122] Indeed, it is self-evident that they do little or nothing to address the health consequences of the occupation, including the death of a 69-year-old Palestinian woman who collapsed and died from a heart attack when Israeli soldiers forced their way into her home and began searching.[123]

In 2005, Palestinian health sector workers signed an open letter that rejected the very premise of cooperation and related initiatives. It states:

> it is more fruitful to consider investing what seems to be a large amount of funds – dedicated by international bodies to such Israeli-Palestinian ventures – directly into Palestinian institutional infrastructure and capacity building, to allow Palestinians to develop the needed human resources, referral services and academic scientific infrastructure that would help them take off on the path of independence and sustainable development. [124]

The letter also warns against 'luring professionals and academics with funds, facilities and opportunities for personal advancement in a resource starved environment, or bringing them solutions to individual medical and systemic problems that the Israeli military occupation of Palestinian land has created and maintained'.[125] The signatories suggested that cooperation would only be justified if it addressed the occupation, which it presented as the 'root cause of ill health' in the territories. In doing so, they showed a clear awareness that Israel's direct control over imports and Palestinian movement is complemented, and to a considerable extent assisted, by a complex system of indirect control that is mediated through constructs of 'development' and 'technical assistance'.

The ability of Palestinian community organizations to resist external pressure was, and continues to be, limited by the various paradoxes and shortcomings produced by the professionalization of Palestinian civil society.[126] The narrow donor focus on service provision, embodied in an abiding fascination with 'outcomes' and 'efficiency', has not been to the benefit of organizations who have historically operated in accordance with very different priorities. The sector has also been adversely impacted by the intrusions of the PA, and more specifically its decrees that regulate NGO activities and inhibit their ability to work in Area C.[127] The situation is even worse in the Gaza Strip, where challenges include isolation from the outside world and protracted 'de-development' (1999: 65).[128]

The health sector's dependence on external donors has therefore been exacerbated by the occupation and the PA's mismanagement. Supposedly neutral donor interventions, which have invariably invoked a host of apolitical technocratic pretexts, have had a profound and long-lasting *political* impact (Khatib et al., 2009: 4).[129]

Here it should be remembered that external donors have in other instances shown a clear reluctance to question, let alone challenge, Israel's colonial activities in the territories (Hanieh, 2008).[130] In 2019, the EU yielded to Israeli pressure and introduced 'anti-terrorism' funding conditions.[131] One year later, it added a new condition to its funding contract, which prohibited NGOs from dealing with individuals that it and Israel regarded as terrorists. The Palestinian NGO Network (PNGO) refused to sign the funding contract and accused the EU of imposing political conditions.[132] If the previous furore over Palestinian textbooks is any guide, the funding of UNRWA schools could well be the next battleground, as Israel has complained that its funding is effectively helping to incite hatred of Israel.[133]

Far from addressing Palestinian health needs, Israel actually has a more established history of seeking to manipulate infectious disease for its own purposes. In 1948, the Haganah poisoned Palestinian water in Acre and Gaza with typhoid germs with the aim of breaking their resistance and producing an epidemic. The Israelis invariably responded to accusations by denying responsibility or blaming a lack of Palestinian hygiene (Pappé, 2006: 100–1).[134]

Salam Abu Sitta (2003) drew on International Committee of the Red Cross (ICRC) files to describe this event in more detail. He notes that 'cast thy bread' or 'donate your bread' (a Hebrew variation of 'give and you get back in return') was linked to a typhoid epidemic in Acre City (in the Gaza Strip) and a cholera epidemic in Egypt and Syria (both in

1948). Sitta observes the Haganah deliberately infected Egyptians and Syrians with cholera with the aim of preventing Arab volunteers from entering Palestine and fighting with Palestinians.[135] In a 2022 article, Benny Morris and Benjamin Ze'ev Kedar drew on Israeli army and Defense Ministry Archives and confirmed these poisoning incidents did occur, and add the operation extended to the Negev, Jericho and Jerusalem. They speak of the operation with considerable sympathy and observe

> The scientists and Haganah/IDF officers probably hoped that they would induce disease, an epidemic even, which would bar militiamen from returning to their villages and attacking Jewish settlements and traffic, reduce the Arabs' ability to prevent Jewish conquest of towns and villages, and create medical havoc among invading Arab troops. As the scientists knew, the availability of antibiotics and vaccines would keep deaths to a minimum (as apparently occurred), but Arab combat effectiveness would be reduced. (Morris and Kedar, 2022: 18)[136]

In the First *Intifada*, it was rumoured that Israel poisoned girls' school water with the aim of sterilizing them. During the First *Intifada*, Israel also used tear gas against Palestinians in closed areas, resulting in deaths. In May 1988, the Federal Laboratories of Pennsylvania announced they would not deliver any more gas to Israel until they received 'some confirmation that their [Israel's] intent [was] not to use it as a weapon' (Rigby, 1991: 61).[137] Given this past history, it is hardly surprising, and is indeed to be expected, that the vaccination rate of Palestinian Jerusalemites will be lower than their Jewish counterparts.[138]

Palestinian health provision in the oPt and the PA's pandemic response

The Palestinian health system was already in a dire state before the pandemic, and this was underlined when a planned strike action was suspended after it broke out. Dr Shawky Sabha, head of the Palestinian medical association, observes: '[I]n 2012 there were 3,300 doctors and in 2019 we had only 2550 doctors, and no staff has been appointed yet.'[139] Meanwhile, the Middle East Monitor observed that '[t]he United States has passed a $900 billion Covid-19 relief bill to support industries and workers affected by the ongoing pandemic, of which hundreds of millions of dollars have been granted to Israel and its defence' (MEMO, 2020).[140] The United States also provided 100 ventilators and a million face masks to Israel in early 2020.[141]

The PA's vaccine distribution has been particularly controversial, in no small part due to its decision to distribute 12,000 vaccine doses to senior PA officials and their families.[142] The Coalition for Accountability and Integrity (AMAN) perhaps had this in mind when it issued a February 2022 statement, in which it warned against the unorganized distribution of vaccinations and emphasized the need for a clear plan that prioritizes high risk groups.[143] This apparent nepotism and favouritism perhaps help to explain why the PA's efforts to establish a *Wakfet Izz* (Dignified Stand) Fund in early April 2020 produced such a tepid and underwhelming response from the Palestinian public.[144] Quite clearly, we should view this as a further illustration of the PA's inability to produce national mobilization in response to ongoing challenges.

The PA's co-option into Israel's colonial strategy, which is consistent with practices of co-option applied elsewhere (Dunbar-Ortiz, 2014: 5),[145] has the clear potential to undermine its Covid-19 strategy. This is important because the elite-popular divide was an important factor in the Ebola Virus Disease (EVD) epidemic in Congo, where it was found that lack of trust in government made people less likely to comply with government guidelines.[146] The same study found that those who 'experienced hardships during the epidemic expressed less trust in government than those who did not, suggesting the possibility of a vicious cycle between distrust, non-compliance, hardships and further distrust'.[147] Colonial activities, including home demolitions and evictions, also make it impossible for Palestinians to follow safety guidelines.[148]

The High Follow-Up Committee, an umbrella organization established in 1982 that represents Palestinian citizens in Israel, responded to official disinterest and inaction by establishing the Arab Emergency Committee, which provides Covid-19 services and guidelines.[149] The inadequacies of the official response have therefore produced civil society mobilization in response.

There are also the physical obstacles that Israel imposes – for example, An-Najah National University Hospital in Nablus, the only university hospital in the oPt that has advanced medical equipment, was prevented from importing a CT scanner.[150] Trump, in an effort to exert pressure on the PA, also cut funding to East Jerusalem hospitals in 2018.[151] This meant that Palestinians were unable to access tertiary care and also undermined health service provision during the pandemic. Israel also attacked three hospitals in the oPt at a time when cases were spiking.[152] The effects of Israel's movement restrictions are also likely to be long-lasting. McNeely et al. observe: 'The consequences of movement restrictions might be even more severe later in life, when the effects of untreated chronic disease become more evident' (2018: 82).[153]

Conclusion

In addressing the contemporary situation in the Palestinian territories, we are not led towards the conclusion that theories of colonialism can contribute important insights and perspectives; rather, we are led to conclude that this is a necessary precondition for understanding and grasping essential contemporary realities. This was once fully understood by the PLO, before this (colonial) insight was consumed by its assorted concessions to political compromise.

We are, however, ultimately drawn to two separate theoretical frameworks, specifically the biopolitical and necropolitical. When combined with an analysis of settler colonial power, both can contribute significant theoretical perspective/s. Biopolitics ruptures an almost intuitive assumption – namely that health intervention seeks to perpetuate and preserve 'life'. On the contrary, Foucault instead reinvents health as part of an expanding spectrum of control and thereby directly implicates it in power relations.

In the territories, Israel's health interventions have, however, historically been limited, and this is characteristic with the general disinterest in the health and well-being of its inhabitants. In contrast to biopolitics, which is networked, multifaceted and dense, the Israeli authorities historically tended to engage with the oPt through somewhat crude and cumbersome military instruments. In the territories at least, the potential of health as a mechanism of political governance therefore remained, to a large extent, essentially unrealized. This has not noticeably changed during the pandemic, as Israel continues to show a steadfast disinterest in the health and well-being of the oPt's inhabitants, even to the point of potentially jeopardizing the health of its own citizens.

Necropolitics, or the 'subjugation of life to the power of death', and the creation of 'death-worlds', more effectively captures key aspects of Israel's relations with the oPt. Necropolitics appears as the exact inverse of biopolitics, in which 'life' is the key referent and justification of intervention; instead, in the case of necropolitics, it is the ability to 'take life' that is foremost and privileged. Death instead appears as an overarching and overpowering presence that gives 'life' a reduced meaning and political significance. Ghanim (2008), however, offers an important insight by proposing thanatopolitics, which is particularly useful because it clarifies that it is the *threat* of death, rather than death itself, that is the foremost political consideration. It is this power to arbitrate on matters of life and death that is integral to the political power that Israel exerts in the oPt. This was clear before the pandemic, but it has been reiterated during the same by various interventions, including efforts to extract maximum political value from the 'leveraging' of essential vaccines and the obstructed movement of essential medical equipment.

Palestinians, however, commit an essential error in looking to the PA for an effective response to the pandemic. In doing so, they fail to acknowledge that, as an essential intermediary in colonial arrangements, it is ill-equipped to provide a leadership role or address the colonial obstacles that continue to impede effective health provision in the oPt. Its failures in the pandemic should not, and indeed cannot be understood in isolation but should instead be attributed to the specific attributes and dysfunctions of its distinctive mode of governance: in other words, this specific failure can only be understood in broader perspective, and by referring to the colonial arrangements that it reproduces and consolidates. Indeed, it would be no exaggeration to assert that the PA is an obstacle to effective health provision rather than a means through which it can be achieved.

Under the terms of the established international consensus, Palestinians are effectively forbidden from drawing this inference and are indeed actively encouraged to engage in various ill-conceived health cooperation projects with Israelis. Through various financial inducements, Palestinians are encouraged to overlook the various ways in which the occupation impedes effective health provision in the territories and directly jeopardizes Palestinian lives. As in other areas of donor intervention, the occupation is effectively 'off-limits'. Such assertions, of course, are diametrically opposed to the political vision of those who stand in opposition to colonial power across the world. This delinking of health issues from the broader political struggle threatens to undermine the basis, meaning and significance of Palestinian resistance: Palestinian medics (who refuse the premise of cooperation initiatives) have clearly grasped this, even if EU policy actors have not. Palestinians continue to resist on the ground and have adapted in response to ongoing health risks. Combating the virus is part of Palestinian resistance and steadfastness in historical Palestine.

Life as death and death as life
The pandemic in the Gaza Strip

During the Oslo secret negotiations, the Israeli prime minister Yitzhak Rabin observed: 'It would be good if Gaza would be swallowed up by the sea, but that's impossible' (quoted in Lustick, 2019: 107[1]). Even before the peace process was established, he therefore clearly established the West Bank and Gaza Strip would be engaged on different terms. Although both are on the basis of the established formula of 'land without people' (Piterberg, 2008; Suárez, 2017).[2]

This of course was not the first or last occasion that Zionism would be forced to adjust to 'unfortunate' or 'inconvenient' realities. Masalha, for example, observes that 'Palestinian demography and the land issue were at the heart of the Zionist transfer mind-set and secret transfer plans of the 1930s and 1940s' (2002: 72; also see Sayegh, 1965: 34).[3] However, the determination of the Arab Palestinian population to 'stay out' ultimately forced it to accept a 'logic of elimination' that was 'not invariably genocidal' (Wolfe, 2006: 387).[4]

Israel's 2005 withdrawal from the Strip, which its political authors went to great lengths to present as a valiant and well-meaning effort to reignite a stagnating peace process, can similarly be understood as a grudging acceptance of established political realities. Pappé more accurately presents it as part of a colonial aspiration towards 'demographic transformation' that can only be understood in historical context. He observes:

> For this reason, the direct control over the Gaza Strip has been abandoned and the Zionist Left supports the two-state solution. But

this course of action is not working and as the recent, more direct ethnic cleansing operations of Israel in the Negev, the Jordan Valley, and the Greater Jerusalem area have shown, the old plan A – of direct expulsion – is still used in order to complete the work that was begun in 1948. (2015: 7)[5]

Indeed, Shimon Peres, Israel's deputy prime minister, explicitly acknowledged that 'demography' was the actual reason for Israel's 'withdrawal',[6] which could more accurately be described as a redeployment in anticipation of future hostilities. And this point is made quite explicitly by Ophir, who observes, '[i]n Gaza, no sovereignty is infringed and no sovereignty is enforced; the withdrawal of state apparatuses has enabled the state to exercise bare force on lives that became bare long ago, without however being engaged in war' (2007: 33).[7] This recalls Veracini's 'non-diplomatic transfer', where 'settler sovereign control of the population's economy was never relinquished' (2010: 45).[8] It is embodied in restrictions of movement, economic sanctions and the denial of trade access to Israel and Egypt. And it includes the creation of 'access restricted areas', including buffer zones on land and limited fishing zones.[9] Al Haq clarifies: 'Most of the buffer zone on land is located on agricultural land while the buffer zone at sea limits fishing activities to an area where fish has already been severely depleted' (2011: 6).[10] And this form of 'transfer' is also embodied in state/peace-building projects after the Second *Intifada* that retained a desire to control and dominate (Bouillon, 2004; Bouris, 2010; Haddad, 2016).[11]

In responding to Hamas's seizure of power in June 2007, Israel imposed a blockade on the Strip and launched wars in 2009, 2012, 2014, 2021 and 2022. Operation Cast Lead (2008–9) killed more than 1,383 Palestinians, including 333 children[12]; Operation Pillar of Defense (2012) killed 173 Palestinians, 38 of whom were children[13]; Operation Protective Edge (2014) killed 2,251 Palestinians, 551 of whom were children.[14] Thousands were injured and require rehabilitation and many children still need psychological help (OCHA, 2014).[15] In the May 2021 aggression, Israel killed 248, including 66 children, and wounded more than 1,900.[16] Fifteen families were wiped out. The Israeli journalist Amira Hass notes 'these were not mistakes' but were approved by high-ranking military officials and jurists. She adds that in the preceding war, more than four times this number (70) of Gazan families were erased under different pretexts.[17] However, rather than confronting Israel over its criminal actions, donors have instead committed to rebuild what it destroyed.[18]

The 'sealing off' of the Strip is not an anomaly or exception, as the 'enclaves' in the West Bank, which are part of an 'exemplary settler colonial project', attest (Lloyd, 2012: 59).[19] And indeed, by as early as 1965, Sayegh was referring to the emergence of 'enclaves' in Israel ('[t]he remnants of Palestine's Arabs who have continued to live in the Zionist settler-state since 1948 have their own "Bantustans", their "native reserves", their "Ghettoes"') (1965: 29).[20] And this was precisely why the Unified National Leadership of the Uprising (UNLU) rejected the principle of autonomy from the outset. In reflecting on its limitations, it observes that 'Palestinian land will remain occupied, settlements will proliferate with generous government support; Israel's army will continue to patrol the streets of Palestinian towns, villages and camps whenever they decide that it is in the interest of the security of Israel' ('Towards a State of Independence', 1988: 245).[21]

Here it is instructive to refer to the autonomy that Menachem Begin outlined during the negotiation of the Camp David peace agreement between Egypt and Israel, which was quite clearly predicated on the understanding that limited freedoms for Palestinians would not imperil Greater Israel (Khalid, 2013: 19–20).[22] Limited Palestinian self-rule in the West Bank and Gaza Strip was therefore tolerable if it did not restrict the rights of Jews to settle in the oPt. Moshe Dayan, the Israeli foreign minister, made this clear in 1979 when he observed that '[Israelis] do not regard ourselves as foreigners in those areas. The Israeli settlements in Judea, Samaria and the Gaza district are there as of right. It is inconceivable to us that Jews should be prohibited from settling and living in Judea and Samaria, which are the heart of our homeland' (Sayegh, 1979: 34).[23]

Here it is instructive to recall the 1993 Cairo Agreement,[24] which established Israel would remain responsible for overall security, including the control of the Strip's 'borders'. Under its terms, redeployed Israeli troops would protect 7,000 settlers who inhabited about a third of Gaza. The remaining two-thirds of the Strip were cantonized and divided between 1.1 million Palestinians, establishing a grossly distorted ratio (128 Israelis for 11,702 Palestinians) in each square mile of the Strip (Roy, 2002: 11).[25]

These and subsequent negotiations were grossly distorted by Israel's security concerns. Aruri explains:

> The section on security consumes about 60 percent of the memorandum, while the rest take up with further redeployment (itself linked to security needs) and unresolved interim issues, including Israeli commitments to negotiate safe passage between the West Bank and Gaza as well as the opening of Gaza airport and eventually a seaport. Extremely brief sections deal with final status talks and 'unilateral actions'. (1999: 18)[26]

However, the enthusiasm with which the PA pursued its 'counter-terrorism' mandate, despite negative consequences (Sayigh, 2009)[27] that included exacerbated internal divisions and democratic deficits,[28] surprised even Uri Savir, Israel's chief negotiator (1998: 102).[29] This clearly recalled Fanon's 'psycho-affective equilibrium', in which the colonized adopts the oppressor's mannerisms and self-image (1963: 210).[30] Accordingly, PA security forces have not merely assisted the colonizer, whether through arbitrary arrests, intelligence gathering or targeted assassinations, but have even imitated the colonizer. This was tragically shown in November 1994 when Palestinian security forces opened fire on Palestinian demonstrators in the Strip, killing thirteen people.

In 2005, Israel unilaterally withdrew from the Strip as part of Sharon's 'disengagement' plan. Escalating internal tensions between Hamas and the PLO erupted two years later when the former violently seized the Strip after disputed 2006 parliamentary elections. As we have seen, the division of the two territories was, however, essentially anticipated by preceding developments, especially in the 'Oslo years'.[31]

In February 2022, the Strip was struck by the fourth and fifth waves of the virus.[32] In early August, Israel arrested Bassam al-Saadi, the senior leader of Islamic Jihad, in Jenin.[33] On 5 August 2022, Israel launched a pre-emptive three-day attack on the Strip that killed 45 Palestinians (including 17 children) and injured more than 300. In return, Islamic Jihad fired hundreds of rockets at Israel. Hamas stood by, after weighing the pros and cons of a war that could weaken its de facto rule.[34] Hamas seems to have accepted the humanitarian and economic incentives that Israel has provided in order to secure a long-term truce. But it cannot entirely disavow the military option,[35] as its commitment to armed resistance legitimizes its rule of the Strip. The fighting was brought to an end by an Egypt-mediated truce.[36] Food prices also rose rapidly in the territory as a result of the Russia-Ukraine War.[37] The economy is still devastated; the health sector remains weak; and patients with chronic illnesses continue to struggle to access hospital services.[38]

Even as I was writing this chapter, the situation in the Gaza Strip further deteriorated as yet another war, the fourth in just over a decade, erupted. Israeli airstrikes hit Hanoun Hospital, Shohada Daraj medical centre, Ministry of Health offices, an orphanage, a female high school, a coronavirus laboratory and the offices of an international relief organization.[39] Roads leading to al-Shifa hospital were also hit.[40] Both primary care services and virus testing were affected, and two medical personnel were also killed (Dr Ayman Abu al-Ouf, head of the internal medicine department and coronavirus response at al-Shifa (the Strip's largest hospital) and Dr Moein Ahmad al-Aloul, one of Gaza's few neurologists, who worked at the same hospital). Dr Jamil Suleiman, from Beit Hanoun, describes the war as the worst war of his fourteen-year experience and describes seeing an entire family wiped out in its early stages.[41]

The wars on Gaza have had a prolonged impact on Gazans and have negatively impacted their basic needs and all aspects of their lives.[42] As Salamanca puts it: 'The modes in which biopower was infused through infrastructure networks to exercise violence over bodies and territory in post-evacuated Gaza, effectively exposed the most ugly face of the radical relationality between colonizer and colonized' (2011: 28).[43] Palestinians are therefore 'bare life' at the mercy of Israel and are, as 'homo sacer', subject to experience death (Agamben, 1998).[44]

These events were clearly anticipated by the attitudes of successive Israeli political elites towards the Strip. In the early 1970s, Ariel Sharon, the then Israeli southern commander divided the Strip, demolished homes and widened roads to allow tanks to enter quarters and neighbourhoods. He also constructed a 53-mile (85km)-long security fence with entry points at Erez, Nahal Oz and Rafah.[45]

From the outset, such actions were framed against a colonial backdrop. Memmi observes that '[c]olonial racism is built from three major ideological components: one, the gulf between the culture of the colonialist and the colonized; two, the exploitation of these differences for the benefit of the colonialist; three, the use of these supposed differences as standards of absolute fact' (1974: 115).[46]

When conceived in this wider perspective, the blockade was not merely the 'natural' consequence of objective processes but was also part of a wider strategy, which included Israel tacitly tolerating the growth of Hamas[47,48] in the hope this would divide the Palestinian national movement (Naser-Najjab and Khatib, 2019: 200).[49] In later years, Benjamin Netanyahu pursued 'divide-and-rule' by allowing Qatar to transfer money to Hamas.[50] However, in 2014, when efforts were being made to establish a unity and reconciliation government, Netanyahu demanded that Mahmoud Abbas decide if he wanted peace with Hamas or Israel. Abbas was abruptly told '[y]ou can have one but not the other'.[51]

When in 2017, the PA cut the salaries of Hamas government public service employees in the Strip (Roy, 2017; Tibon, 2018),[52] it was widely seen as the latest development in an internal Palestinian power struggle.[53] However, here it should be remembered that the Palestine Papers, which Al Jazeera released in 2011, revealed that the PA had, during the course of negotiations in the period 1999–2010, actually *encouraged* Israel to impose even harsher measures on the Strip (Swisher, 2011: 53–71).[54] The PA and the 'international community' have also accepted Israel's labelling of the Strip, which justifies different applications of force to the Strip, including the use of vaccines as a bargaining tool.[55]

In retrospect, therefore, withdrawal was not a concession to peace but was instead intended to place the Strip beyond the limits of the permissible. As Salamanca explains, '[t]he categorization of Gaza as an "enemy entity" is a clear-cut example of the way the machinery of *imaginative geographies* [emphasis in original] is put into motion and how it is used to justify the cuts and disruptions of infrastructure networks as a measure of collective punishment' (2011: 28).[56] And here it is instructive to recall Badarin's observation that the 'othering' relationship 'is sustained through a process of differentiation that first constructed the "other" (Hamas and Gaza) as a security concern and source of danger. It was therefore necessary to extricate this "other" from the assumed "self"' (2016: 163).[57]

In the Strip, Israel is able to exercise necropolitical power over Palestinians who are dehumanized and condemned to endure an 'animal life' (Mbembe, 2003: 24).[58] During thirteen years of siege Israel deployed different weapons 'in the interest of maximum destruction of persons and the creation of death-worlds' (Mbembe, 2003: 40).[59] In buffer zones, for example, Israel defines the boundaries of 'access restricted' areas where Palestinians are killed or injured.[60]

Given that there has historically been a reluctance to acknowledge the apartheid or colonial character of Israel, it should not occasion surprise that accusations of genocide have been similarly viewed as unacceptable or impermissible. Here it is worthwhile to consider Israel's control of the territory's fuel supply and more precisely the way it is (mis)used to collectively punish Gazans.[61] And, in doing so, acknowledge that Fanon's interpretation of occupation closely resembled genocide. He observes: 'There is not occupation of territory on the one hand and independence of persons on the other. It is the country as a whole, its history, its daily pulsation that are contested, disfigured, in the hope of a final destruction. Under these conditions, the individual's breathing is an observed, an occupied breathing. It is a combat breathing' (1994: 65).[62]

And this also seems to be implied by Abujidi, who refers to the Strip as the '[s]tate of Urbicide that presents the extreme condition of the State of Siege' and clarifies '[t]he State of Urbicide is the permanent state of invasion, destruction and extreme strangulation taking place in many Palestinian cities and refugee camps within the State of Occupation and Siege' (2009: 275).[63] Gazans are, to borrow a phrase of Fanon's, 'hemmed in' (Fanon, 1963: 52).[64] The Strip is one of the most densely populated places in the world, bringing to mind Fanon's allusion to 'a world without spaciousness [where] men live [on] top of each other' (1963: 39).[65]

Genocide is indiscriminate and here it should be remembered that Israel's blockade bans dual-use items that are primarily used for civilian purposes but could also be adapted for military purposes. However, the definitions that Israel applies are not clear and are arbitrary and open to interpretation.[66]

The Israeli Ministry of Health calculated a calorie count on the basis of age and gender with the aim of limiting the amount of food that would be allowed to enter the Strip and did this with the intention of 'allow[ing] for a basic fabric of life' (Gisha, 2012: 5).[67] In 2008, Israel told the United States that it would seek to bring Gaza's economy to the 'brink of collapse' while 'avoiding a humanitarian crisis' by allowing it to 'function at the lowest level possible'.[68] The blockade clearly recalls Mbembe's fate of the 'living dead', who are always confronted by death (2003: 40).[69]

As Winter correctly observes, '[h]umanitarianism is therefore not a direct challenge to the siege but [is] part of its functioning mechanism' (2016: 314).[70] Furthermore, '[w]hile the siege does not annihilate the population, it turns welfare, nutrition, health, and security into vectors of punishment and coercion' (2016: 313).[71] While it is implemented over time and is to this extent consistent with 'sieges [that] are marked by a slow and protracted temporality; the coercion does not condensate in a single, temporally compacted event but is dispersed and drawn out, reaching its effect only cumulatively' (Winter 2016: 310).[72]

Donors and the 'international community' are directly implicated not just by their actions, but also by their inactions. Abu Sittah further elaborates: 'After every war on Gaza, donor conferences raise billions of dollars to rebuild infrastructure. Despite the inevitability that Israel will destroy Gaza again.' And he adds that this '[h]umanitarianism dehistoricizes and depoliticizes the conflict by reducing it to balance sheets of human suffering' (2020: 15).[73]

And adds: 'The siege allows Israel to shift the discourse around Gaza from one of national liberation, occupation, and self-determination to the balance sheet of humanitarian aid: the numbers of trucks allowed in, hours of electricity, the amount of medical supplies, and the number of patients allowed out for treatment' (2020: 15).[74] Even when the PA sent vaccine doses to Gaza in September 2021, Israel's security checks delayed the shipment and then obliged the Ministry of Health to destroy 50,000 doses (MAP, 2022: 5).[75] But it is still worse than this – the wars in the Strip have provided a testing ground for Israeli weapons[76] and have enabled it to market its armaments[77] and became established as 'the world's largest exporter of drones'.[78]

In the Strip, life has therefore degraded to the point where it is without meaning or purpose. In 2017, the United Nations reported, three years before the outbreak of the pandemic, that the Strip's debilitated infrastructure and grossly degraded living circumstances would make it 'unliveable' by 2020.[79] A year later, the May 2021 war on the Strip, aggravated the situation even further. [80]

For Western observers currently struggling to remember what life was like before the pandemic, it might seem perverse to consider it being regarded as an inconvenience one among a number of ongoing challenges. Nonetheless, this is the case in the Strip, where successive wars and the ongoing degradation of basic living conditions (two-thirds of Gazans are food insecure)[81] have created a kind of fatalism and an associated resignation to the force of ongoing events. Gazans can quite clearly see that the virus is not the reason for the lack of services, high unemployment and absence of future opportunities.

Amjad Yaghi, a young journalist, told me:

Corona is not more dangerous than the blockade. The blockade has a negative impact at all levels, social, economy, politics. Young injured

Gazans suffer from power cuts, for example. They are unable to tolerate the heat with implanted Platinum Metals and Prostheses. They take into the streets seeking breeze. We used to say, streets are full of crippled.

And added:

Most youth are workers on daily bases with no permanent contracts. Some of them work in cafes and restaurants at the beach. During closure, either no jobs or less hours, the government did not compensate them. These workers have no rights. Jobs are day to day. There is a huge psychological stress, but no appropriate mental health support is available. Also, mental health support won't work because situation is the same.[82]

Almost two-thirds of the Strip's population are below twenty-five years of age. They live without hope and future prospects. Yara (not her real name) observes: 'People tell me we don't want to live. It is because of the situation, they love life but they want a different one. Some people never travelled by plane, never been to cinema, or theatre, they see these things on TV, when electricity is available.'[83]

This is echoed by Dr Abed, who told me that 'there is hopelessness and lack of confidence. Many people told me that people do not die from Corona but would die from hunger and siege'.[84] Some interviewees, including Dr Abed, however, claimed that the siege delayed the spread of the virus for seven months. Under these conditions, distinctions between rich and poor, and associated entitlements and privileges, have evaporated.[85] In this living hell, all are condemned to the same fate.

Rawia Hamam, the direction of training and scientific research department at Gaza Community Mental Health Programme (GCMHP),[86] similarly asserts that the coronavirus is not the main concern for Gazans. She explains:

When my family and I were watching the news of the first corona cases among the community in Gaza, many other things were happening. An Israeli drone was flying, a young man committed suicide, an explosion in Shujaiya, (internal explosion, by accident), power cut at 10.00 [electricity runs for 4 hours a day]. Israel tightening the blockade, the

Egyptian mediation to deescalate tension failed.[87] My children asked us why did you bring us to this world?

She also relates a story from the Strip in 15 September 2020:

> During the period of normalisation agreements between August and September 2020 between Arab countries (United Arab Emirates (UAE), Bahrain, and Sudan and Israel. It was while hearing sounds of explosions, a father asks his 13 year son to open the windows to avoid the pressure and fall of the window. His son replied, 'we are fed up with the blockade and the Corona, we want war to die. We do not want to live half dead. We live in hell, it can't be that God is punishing us to send us later to heaven'.

Ahmad (not his real name), an academic whose work focuses on nursing and psychology,[88] told me that '[a] generation born 2002 witnessed 3 wars (now four wars) killed more people than Corona . . . they adapted to death. In the latest march of return Israel killed more than 200 Palestinians, injured 8,000; [and created] more than 156 amputated, [who] need rehabilitation' (see OCHA, 2020a).[89]

It is therefore essential to recognize the extent to which respect for human life in the Strip has already degraded. During the marches of return, Israeli snipers openly admitted they deliberately targeted the knees of protesting Palestinians.[90] Puar observes that '[m]aiming as intentional practice expands biopolitics beyond simply the question of "right of death and power over life"' (2015: 6). And adds that '[m]aiming masquerades as "let live" when in fact it acts as "will not let die"'(2015: 8).[91] In this instance, we refer to power *over* life rather than the power to *take* life.

The Strip's degraded healthcare system

One year after Covid-19 first broke out, Israel has managed to vaccinate half of its population, as cases in the Strip continued to spike.[92] Lina (not her real name),[93] a health professional interviewee who wished to remain anonymous, told me that 'Gaza is mostly refugees [who] live in the camps with extended families, which makes social distancing difficult. However, many coronavirus deaths are due to pre-existing conditions. The infrastructure is ineffective and poverty rate is high.' Despite this, Israel prohibited 2,000 vaccination doses from entering the Strip, at a time when cases were spiking.[94]

The problems that are now being experienced can therefore be traced back to the preceding period and, more specifically, the blockade, which has destroyed the Strip's health infrastructure. Lina (not her real name) observes that the impact of the siege is more grave than the virus and claims that 'if you compare deaths before corona and now the numbers are higher before the pandemic'.

The OCHA has also observed that the pandemic has resulted in an increase in the number of youth suicides.[95] This was confirmed by most interviewees.[96] Lina (not her real name) explains that '[t]here are suicide cases among youngsters, but Hamas report them as accidents. These youngsters finish education but no jobs.'[97]

Rawia[98] also explains that, 'suicide cases are increasing but are not recorded. Most of these young people have no jobs. Unemployment is leading these young people to feeling of hopelessness. There are people who graduated in 2011, most of them are now in their thirties. When they apply for training programs in 2020, we realize that for ten years they did nothing.'

She adds:

> The pandemic, compounded by double lockdowns, created the conditions for fears and worries, distress and anxieties to rise among all, with effects on mental health of different age groups and genders, particularly frontline health staff, women, young children, wage and salaried workers, and university students.[99]

Youngsters' feeling of hopelessness and despair is deepening and they are unable to see a way out. Saleh Abu Shamala,[100] a 28-year-old from Rafah, told me:

> My friends and I used to believe of the possibility of change, now it is about individuals. Things get worse and youngsters live in despair, some

commit suicide or decide to live day-by-day. The siege is suffocating us, last time I travelled was 3 years ago, I had an internship. It took me four months to complete papers. You need a security clearance from Israel, which takes 70 working days. It is expensive to travel, to cross Rafah crossing, you need to pay 1400 USD, any delays on your way to Egypt, will lead to missing the flight forcing one to book a hotel room and pay additional cost. We believed in a collective project, now it is about a personal project, it is about either getting married, have children and live without ambition and goals or find a way to leave Gaza, some join political parties to get salaries.

Rawia also highlights an important gender dimension, noting that although there are hotlines available, women rarely call, despite the fact that under lockdown violence against them has increased. As economic constraints have tightened, they have also had to take on more responsibility for immediate and extended family. Men call hotlines and complain about debts and poverty, and their inability to provide food to their children.[101]

When the United States cut its funding to UNRWA[102] in 2018, it undermined the Strip's primary health system and the ability of its impoverished population[103] to confront the pandemic (Abed, 2020: 4)[104] The pre-pandemic situation in the Strip, including an inadequate sewage system, lack of clean water and electricity shortages,[105] also created an environment where Covid-19 could thrive. As Alkhaldi explains: '[B]eing poor means living conditions are unhealthy and overcrowded, access to clean water and good food is non-existent, and buying disinfectants, gloves and masks is unaffordable' (2020: 1247).[106] Israel has also halted the issuing of permits to patients with chronic illnesses who require treatment in Israel and the West Bank or who require international medical care.[107]

The blockade, which has made it difficult to repair or replace damaged facilities or equipment and also produces shortages of medicines, is the foremost obstacle that has impeded basic standards of medical provision in the Strip. Patients with pre-existing conditions also lack care. The treatment of patients with chronic illnesses has been suspended because of resource limitations and the prioritization of Covid patients.[108] Israel controls the registration of patients and is responsible for issuing IDs that determine official status, (Gisha, 2011: 128)[109] and the associated restrictions that it has imposed have made it difficult for patients from the Strip to seek medical treatment abroad.

Those who seek this are required to demonstrate 'good conduct', which involves providing documents, obtaining travel permission and, in some cases, 'informing' in return for permits.[110] However, the impact of successive wars should also be taken into account: Israel has destroyed or damaged ambulances, hospitals and primary healthcare centres, and has also attacked, injured or killed medical and health workers. Tawil-Souri has spoken of a 'regime of digital occupation' (2012: 28) that has limited Gazans' 'integration into the network' (2012: 35)[111] and hindered their ability to respond to the pandemic.

The Strip has fourteen hospitals, fifty Ministry of Health primary care clinics and twenty-two UNRWA clinics,[112] But they are poorly equipped and lack medicines. They were barely able to meet minimum health needs before the pandemic but are now confronted by challenges of unimaginable scope. Dr Fathi Abuwarda, the advisor to the minister of health, speaking only a few months after the outbreak of the pandemic, observes: 'We have entered the catastrophe stage and if we continue like this, the healthcare system will collapse.' And he adds: 'The best solution is a full lockdown for 14 days, which will allow medical teams to control and combat the virus, with only shops that provide food supplies kept open.'[113]

The 2014 war directly impacted the Strip's (already poor) health system and ability to act in accordance with WASH (Water, Sanitation and Health) best practices.[114] A 2019 B'Tselem report observed that '[a]bout 18,000 residential units were either completely destroyed or heavily damaged, leaving more than 100,000 Palestinians – some 17,000 families – homeless.'[115]

The health sector was severely damaged by attacks that damaged hospitals, rehabilitation centres and ambulances, and killed medical workers.[116] Medical workers were also hit hard during the Great

Return March, which began on 30 March 2018, and was intended to commemorate the seventieth anniversary of the Nakba. Three were killed, and 845 were injured. And 112 ambulances and seven health services were destroyed.

Hamas and its pandemic response

Hamas initially imposed very strict measures in an attempt to avoid catastrophe. Dr Yehya Abed explains,[117]

> We imposed restrictions. We used the siege and imposed a very strict lockdown. Even when the Palestinian Health minister asked us to exempt two ministers from quarantine to visit Gaza, we refused. The quarantine was for 21 days because it was the beginning and we did not have enough information. We used schools for quarantine, hotels owners offered to use their venues, which enhanced conditions of quarantine. Later we built 1000 rooms (500 in the north and 500 in the south). It was mostly voluntary efforts. Thus, for 7 month there was not a single case. During this period, we became better informed about the virus. For example, at that time we had no facilities for tests, WHO took samples to Ramallah for testing.

These and other measures helped to ensure that no positive cases were recorded in the Strip in an initial seven-month period (Abu-Oudah et al., 2021).[118]

Dr Abed observes:

> This period enabled us to establish facilities. For seven months, we were busy preparing services across the strip. We prepared European Hospital was fully prepared for COVID (240 beds) and we received ventilators. Turkish Hospital[119] helped us…there were some issues with Turkey because it prepared the hospital without human resources or running cost, thus, inauguration took a long time it needed minister of health and Turkey approval. Due to the pandemic, we got the approval. In any case, most cases were mild or asymptotic.

The Palestinian Health and Interior ministries provided daily updates on tests, cases and deaths, and the general public improvised by producing their own personal protective equipment (PPE), including masks (Abu-Oudah et al., 2021: 47).[120] Vaccine distribution was generally viewed as fair, although this probably reflected the fact they were distributed by UNRWA.[121] Public take-up of the vaccine has, however, been limited. There are also ongoing shortages of basic medicines, including paracetamol. This affects even those who have insurance,[122] with the result that many are forced to resort to private health care.[123]

Hamas's initial commitment to strong preventative measures rooted in a public health response appears to be subsided, and Rawia claims that it has lifted lockdown restrictions in response to popular pressures. This was shown during Laylat al-Qadr, or the Night of Destiny, the most sacred in the Muslim holy month of Ramadan, in mosques across the Strip, when there was no social distancing.[124]

This is just one example of the corruption of Hamas, which has become unavoidable; it was remarked on by most interviewees, some of whom even claimed that Hamas was only saved by the recent war.[125] Social media and activist criticism also increased the pressure on Hamas, with the result that it eased a number of social restrictions, such as forcing women to wear the hijab.

Ahmad notes this change in Hamas's positions and provides historical context by referring to its previous contacts with the UN and some EU member states.[126] In 2012, Taher Nouno, the Hamas spokesperson, said: 'We want a direct dialogue with European leaders so that they can hear from us, not just to hear about us.' And added: 'This dialogue is very important. Maybe we can change our minds on some issues and maybe European countries can change their minds on some issues.'[127]

According to the *Guardian* EU representatives, including Britain, secretly met with Hamas leaders in 2013[128] and this may have influenced developments during the most recent war in the Strip, when EU–US divide emerged on the possibility of a ceasefire and Middle Eastern issues more generally.[129] Yara (not her real name) suggests this is part of an attempt by Hamas to project a more positive, pro-democratic, image onto the world. She observes:

> Once Yehiya Sinwar, (the present Hamas leader, elected in 2017) invited civil society organisations to discuss. This was late 2019. I told Sinwar that this meeting is self-serving, a show off, to appear liberal to donors and to Mahmoud Abbas that you discuss the general elections with civil society. If you take me as a partner, we need to be part of everything. He was tolerant and listened, but in reality Hamas arrests opposition activists. One time I followed a case of an activist arrested. I told a prosecutor that a person was arrested without warrant, he replied, 'I am the law here'.

In response to these and other developments, the 'international community' has also made it clear, including after the most recent war, that it is unwilling to provide aid that could benefit Hamas. For example, Yehiya Sinwar committed, during a press conference, that Hamas would not 'take a single cent intended for reconstruction and humanitarian efforts'.[130]

Continued opposition to Hamas also reflects the group's excessive taxes and control of the Sinai tunnels.[131] This is echoed by a Transparency International anti-corruption report that observes how the occupation and political division have aggravated corruption in the oPt. In noting how both 'sides' have sought to increase their power, it reflects on how this has led to '[a] lack of transparency of public institutions and public fund management, and low trust in public institutions' (Schoeberlein, 2019: 13).[132]

In early 2019, Gazans took to the streets to protest against corruption and oppression, and afterwards complained that Hamas had responded with excessive violence.[133] Other interviewees accused Hamas of manipulating popular protests (the March of Return) for its own purposes. Saleh Abu Shamala[134] said:

> Protests started a year after the movement of 'we want to live' campaign was established against raising taxes. Hamas arrested people and brutally supressed them. The idea of March of Return was a peaceful

and activists were non-violent at the beginning. Hamas encouraged people to participate to cross Karem Abu Salem and destroy it. PA ended up paying for repair.[135] For Hamas, March of return was a source of funding although many of the injured were not compensated to cover expenses of their treatments.

One father, who had to treat his own son, directed his criticism towards Hamas. He said: 'Let the heads of the Hamas come and see my son, only yesterday they received the Qatari money[136], and what did they do with it? They split the money among themselves.'[137]

Ahmad affirms that Hamas discriminates in favour of its supporters when distributing aid. And Lina alleges it artificially inflates Covid-19 to obtain funding. Nepotism, personal benefits (both in the form of business and donations) and financial support for Hamas hospitals and clinics all show how Hamas conducts itself as a political party, and not as a government.[138]

Since 2007, when Hamas seized power in Gaza, internal division has defined Palestinian political life. 'Public' employment emerged as a feature of this divide. Clarno observes: 'Like Israel, the PA also uses public employment as a pressure release valve. Since 2007, the PA has renewed its commitment to free-market economics yet continues to rely on public sector jobs to contain unemployment and resistance' (2017: 105).[139]

The PA has therefore politicized the employment of civil servants in accordance with the stated wishes of the international community,[140] with the result that it has become part of the Fatah-Hamas power struggle. In the period after 2007, the PA in Ramallah asked civil servants not to report to work under the Hamas government, and committed to continue to pay their salaries. At the end of 2013, EU auditors challenged this arrangement.[141] But this was questioned by Peter Stano, spokesperson for the European Commission, who said: 'If the Palestinian Authority is not paying these people, who is going to provide for them?' Stano said, 'If you have people running around without income, they are more prone to be taken by extremism, by forces we have no contact with.'[142] Aside from anything else, this again reiterated the extent to which the siege of the Strip proceeds in accordance with international designs, and functions as part of the neoliberal order.[143]

By this time, the salaries of 38,000 civil servants in Gaza had been cut or not paid for months. In 2017, the PA forcibly retired thousands of Gazan employees and cut 30 per cent of the remaining salaries, after accusing Hamas of failing to transfer tax revenues. And in the following year, it halved the salaries of Gazans or did not transfer them at all.[144] Qatar paid the salaries of 40,000 civil servants. In 2019, further cuts were imposed after Israel withheld tax revenues after refusing to pay the salaries of Palestinian prisoners. Although the PA continued to pay the full salaries of West Bank civil servants, the pandemic forced it to impose cuts.[145]

Most interviewees spoke about the economic impact of the geopolitical division of the West Bank and Gaza Strip. Ahmad explains that '[p]eople in Gaza are more concerned about the division that affects economy. The salary cuts for 4 years. I get only 40% of my salary while staying at home (there are 3000 of the 8000 employees of ministry of higher education'.[146] Mohamed Ramadan adds:

> It is not fair to say that COVID 19 is the cause of the bad situation in Gaza. The situation is difficult since 2007. We live under exceptional situation as Israel considered Gaza a hostile entity . . . everything is in halt, restriction of movement, economic crisis, no production and so on. These Israeli policies forces us to only think of basic needs.

He told me that, in general, employees in Gaza suffer, he explains, 'In hospitals, employees get 40% of basic salary, average $300, they have fixed contracts, with no rights or pension.'[147]

Interviewees also spoke of how the blockade had affected the Strip's electricity supply, accusing Hamas of exploiting people by forcing them to pay triple the price. In the Strip, power is provided by Israel, Egypt and a fuel-based power plant[148] that is only maintained with the acquiescence of Israel, the PA and Egypt. Even when this is forthcoming, Gazans only receive a few hours of electricity.

Mohamed Ramadan[149] observes that 'given the low salaries and unemployment, not many people can afford [electricity]. Even when fuel cost is covered by Egypt or Qatar, it is resold to people. I have an air condition unit, but do not use, I do not want to get used to it, given the unpredictable power cuts.'

One of the (anonymous) interviewees claimed that electricity provision was all about money laundering and that government institutions received electricity for free. Yara[150] adds:

> The recent war destroyed the infrastructure we now have only 3 hour of electricity and no water. In Gaza electricity and internet, the most expensive in the world. External generators are owned by people close to Hamas they take it from the municipality, they now created committee for these sellers to legalise it. When people protested, Hamas government tried to lower the price, owner turned the generators off in 2020. Tried to reach an agreement with the government, but nothing materialised.[151]

Donor funding criteria has affected aid to Gaza, and several (especially the United States) imposed various conditions, including not employing members or supporters of Hamas. Humanitarian and development work became 'securitized' as a result,[152] and Israeli definitions of terrorism contributed to this.[153]

Dr Yehya Abed shared his experience of donors in the Strip:

> I was director of research in health ministry and worked with USAID on two projects . . . every funding is conditional . . . most funding is not about development, only basic needs and relief. Any project not based on relief, is ignored, building factories for example.[154] [And added] Although USAID and UNRWA cut funding, which affected health system negatively, donations increased from Gulf states during corona that enabled us to build diagnostic facilities, lab facilities. We have enough beds, never had shortage . . . no shortage in oxygen, they sent Oxygen, synthetizing products.[155]

On 28 May 2021, the Palestine Forum organized a closed event, which I attended,[156] which gave Gazan activists, all of whom were anonymous in order to ensure their security, a chance to share their views and experiences. In the event, Hamas was criticized for using the war for its own political purposes, and for ignoring civilian loss of life and damage to infrastructure. The sentiments of many were encapsulated when one participant said 'we live day to day, with no plans for the future'. Another contributor addressed the blockade, noting 'the blockade is worse now than before the war and we are starting from zero in terms of basic good allowed in. There is restriction on basic food and goods now' (see OCHA, 2021)).[157] Another referred to the central challenge confronting Gazans, noting 'our problem is not humanitarian or reconstruction; homes can be rebuilt, but it is about dignity, freedom and justice' (see World Bank, 2017).[158]

Conclusion

In Western democracies, Covid-19 is a threat to life and this vividly contrasts with the Strip, where it is a threat to a life that does not exist or to a 'life' more akin to a living death. Here the pandemic is not elevated above all else but is placed below more immediate considerations, including the ongoing blockade and continued Palestinian political divisions.

This situation, which will no doubt seem perverse to Western readers, shows just how far the value of life has degraded in the Strip. Various parties are responsible for this, including the PA, Hamas, and of course, Israel. From the perspective of Gazans who have come to question the very meaning of life, the emergence of yet another threat is just one more factor to take into account.

It should also be recognized that the pandemic is effectively superimposed on pre-existent injustices and privations. The pandemic is, in other words, only experienced through the continued blockade, the inhuman legacy of four successive, endemic human rights violations, huge unemployment and continued internal division. For Gazans, it is effectively meaningless to speak of the pandemic without first referring to these factors.

The formal recognition that Israel ostensibly extends to the PA is not granted to Gazans who, as 'bare life', can be disposed of without a second thought or consideration. From Rabin, who openly willed Gaza's disappearance into the sea, to his successors, who have happily endorsed the indiscriminate slaughter of whole families as state policy, Israel's leaders have never tried to conceal their apparently limitless contempt for the people of the Strip. And it is here, where over two-thirds of the population are refugees or descendants of refugees, where Israel's continued failure to acknowledge, let alone address, questions of historical justice is most starkly demonstrated.

Wolfe has previously spoken of a 'logic of elimination' that was 'not invariably genocidal'. (2006: 387).[159] However, in the case of the Strip, where Israel has obstructed the passage of essential medical supplies and effectively denied Palestinians access to life-saving medical treatment, we are obliged to ask if this distinction still holds and if we are confronted by something that more closely, in crucial aspects and dimensions, resembles and recalls genocide.

Reflecting on the pandemic in the Strip, we can react in many ways, but not with surprise, for the precise reason that it would be more perverse if the Israeli authorities, having assiduously pursued a murderous campaign of dehumanization should suddenly, in response to the pandemic, decide to grant Gazans the status and associated entitlements it had hitherto so completely and consistently denied. And we should similarly not react with shock or surprise when we encounter a 'logic of elimination' that consistently seeks to deny Gazans a meaningful existence and that inflicts a 'bare life' on them.

In the Strip, as in the West Bank, a 'double occupation' frustrates the possibility of future development and progress. Given this, it is hardly surprising that Covid-19 is not the main or most pressing priority for Gazans. Instead, the imperative of resistance, which requires a unified will and purpose as a prerequisite, is viewed as the greater priority. In this deeply politicized environment, where the conditions of Palestinian suffering are clearly linked to political decisions taken or not taken, political organization and mobilization instead appear as the pre-eminent priorities. The alternative is a surrender to 'bare life', despair and inaction.

Bare apartheid

The pandemic in Hebron

Hebron is the largest Palestinian city in the West Bank after Jerusalem, with an estimated population of more than 221,000 (Hebron Governorate has an estimated population of 760,000).[1] Israeli surveillance and repression in Hebron City, including checkpoints, closures and an Israeli 'gaze' that combines technological and settler surveillance, have reduced it to a 'ghost town' (2015: 5).[2] There is an Israeli settlement in the centre, where about 600 settlers are protected by around 2,000 Israeli soldiers. This number is currently set to double.[3]

As in Jerusalem, the colonial settlement of Hebron began almost immediately after the end of the Six-Day War. In 1968, a few ultra-Orthodox Jewish families who were led by Rabbi Moshe Levinger went to Hebron's Park Hotel with the apparent intention of observing Passover. After arriving, they informed the Israeli government they would never leave. The Israeli government, and most notably the defence minister Moshe Dayan, accepted their demands and allowed them to stay and establish the Kiryat Arba (the City of Four) settlement.[4] A recent document shows that Israel invoked military and security pretexts to build settlements, including Kiryat Arba, on privately owned land, with the aim of circumventing international law's prohibition on transferring civilians to occupied land.[5] A secret document that was declassified in 2016 explained that the mayor of Hebron would be informed that the Israeli army had begun building 'houses on the military base in preparation for winter'.[6] After the settlement was completed, Moshe Dayan announced, in a July 1973 interview, that '[t]here is no more Palestine. Finished' (quoted in Shlaim, 2000: 321).[7]

From the outset, the Israeli government was aware it had no right to establish civilian settlements on occupied land (2000: 321).[8] However, this did not stop Yigal Allon, the then deputy prime minister, from putting forward the 'Allon Plan', which proposed annexing Jerusalem, the Jordan Valley and areas around Hebron (Raz, 2012: 244–7).[9] The Plan continues to influence Israeli policy and settlements have become established as part of a surveillance system that controls Palestinian land and space (Weizman, 2007 and Halper, 2015).[10]

Thousands of Palestinians have been displaced from the centre of the city since the first settlement was built in the 1970s. Emad Hamdan, the director of the Hebron Rehabilitation Committee, observes: '[t]oday, in 2016, there are about 6,500 Palestinians who reside in the area. On a daily basis, they live with the imminent threat of being attacked, harassed, displaced or killed. I estimate that the population is 60 percent less than what it would have been if there was no occupation and settlers' (BADIL, 2016: 9).

After Kiryat Arba was finished, Hebron became a target for continuous colonization. In 1979, the Beit Hadassah building was occupied by settlers. At the end of 2019, the Israeli government announced it was building a new settlement in the old city on land owned by the municipality, which would replace a wholesale market that Palestinians were banned from accessing since the 25 February 1994 massacre, when the Jewish-American settler Baruch Goldstein opened fire on praying Palestinian Muslims, killing twenty-nine and injuring more than a hundred.[11] In castigating these and other restrictions imposed on the city in the name of 'security', Palestinians bitterly complained that the victims were being punished for Goldstein's crimes.[12]

After the massacre, Israel closed the mosque for six months and then divided it into Muslim and Jewish prayer sections, and continued to restrict Palestinian access. It also prevented Palestinians from accessing Shuhada Street, which had previously been an important economic hub in the city. In referring to the consequences of this (continued) closure, OCHA (2013) observes:

The harsh access restrictions have forced the vast majority of Palestinians living along [Shuhada] street to abandon their homes and be displaced elsewhere. The few families that remained face difficult living conditions. While some of them are exceptionally allowed to use a small section of the street to enter their homes, other families must rely on back entrances, or their neighbours' rooftops to enter their homes. As a result, otherwise normal activities, such as bringing home foodstuff or furniture, became complicated operations; receiving visitors became almost prohibitive.[13]

In the Second *Intifada,* Israel issued twenty-one military orders in the Old City that displaced 6,000 residents and resulted in the immediate closure of about 2,500 shops and businesses by 2003.[14] Military zone areas in and around the city remain 'off-limits' to Palestinians.

The apartheid reality drives displacement.[15] By 1996, the Palestinian population in the Old City had decreased by almost 75 per cent, falling from 1,501 to 400 (BADIL, 2016: 85).[16] In acknowledging the challenges that continued to confront Palestinians in the city, Yasser Arafat issued a presidential decree in August 1996 that created the Hebron Rehabilitation Committee (HRC), which supported Palestinians in Hebron's old city with the aim of encouraging them to stay. The Committee helped renovate houses and planned projects that would improve living conditions and create jobs.[17] However, its important work was repeatedly frustrated by Israel's building and construction permit requirements.[18]

Hebron was exempt from the Oslo II arrangements for urban areas, including Bethlehem, Jenin, Nablus, Ramallah and Tulkarm, that were introduced in 1995. The subsequent election of Benyamin Netanyahu as Israel's prime minister in May 1996 did not have as significant an impact on the peace process as might be presumed, precisely because there is such a thin dividing line between Israeli 'Hawks' and 'Doves' (Mharib, 1971: 17)[19]. And indeed, Netanyahu continued to negotiate with the PLO on unresolved issues, including Israel's redeployment from Hebron.[20] The Hebron Protocol, which was signed on 17 January

1997, established the basis for a limited Israeli redeployment from Hebron. It divided the city into two areas (H1 and H2) and established the Israeli army would protect Israeli settlers in H2 areas (JPS, 1997: 131),[21] where 800 Israeli settlers live among 34,000 Palestinians.[22] This mixed model is similar to arrangements in rural areas of the West Bank – Dr Hazem Ashhab observes that '[i]n some villages the center is Area A, under full Palestinian authority, and the rest is Area B. Within these villages, however, there are areas B and C.'[23]

The Protocol did not just seek to maintain the status quo but also sought to create 'facts on the ground'. Sayegh explains that '[w]hile the instruments of colonisation were being laboriously created, diplomatic efforts were also being exerted to produce *political conditions* (emphasis in original) that would permit, facilitate, and protect large-scale colonisation' (1965: 6).[24] Netanyahu reiterated this in a statement to the Knesset in January 1997. He said: 'We do not want to remove the Jewish community from Hebron. We want to preserve and consolidate it. We do not want to remove ourselves from Hebron; we want to remain in Hebron' (JPS, 1997: 142).[25] He wanted to negotiate the Hebron redeployment separately, and to 'delink' it from the peace process and unresolved issues (Andoni, 1997: 19).[26] However, he also used the Hebron negotiations to redefine Oslo II. The United States accepted Israel's definition of security and did not seek to amend statements in the Protocol's annex (JPS, 1997: 138–9),[27] and this was why Israel's security was prioritized, both during the redeployment in Hebron and the West Bank more generally.

Lamis Andoni observes 'that the security arrangements were designed to ensure nonfriction between the Palestinian and the Israeli in the long term', and adds the arrangements in Hebron, according to Clinton administration officials, were intended to provide 'an example of future coexistence between the PA and settlers throughout the West Bank and the Gaza Strip' (1997: 24).[28]

The Protocol established that '[t]here will be a redeployment of Israeli military forces in the city of Hebron except for places and roads where they are necessary for the security and protection of Israelis and their movement'. (JPS, 1997: 131).[29] Article 9 of the Protocol states:

> Both sides reiterate their commitment to the unity of the City of Hebron, and their understanding that the division of security responsibility will not divide the city. [...] both sides share the mutual goal that movement of people, goods and vehicles within and in and out of the city will be smooth and normal, without obstacles or barriers. (JPS, 1997: 134)[30]

The settlements, which enable Israel to extensively project its power across the city (and most notably the Old City), affect all aspects of Palestinian life and also impact all Palestinians, including schoolchildren. In seeking to protect the settlers, Israel has established twenty-two checkpoints, built more than sixty barriers and created closed military zones. Palestinians are arbitrarily arrested and administratively detained, without charges.[31] Children are also arrested and interrogated without a responsible adult being present.[32]

Here, Israel imposes arbitrary laws that leaves Palestinians in a constant 'state of exception'. The juridical order is suspended and replaced by violence (Agamben, 2005: 4),[33] while controls are extended as a kind of 'biopolitics of population' that is meant to discipline and subjugate Palestinians (Foucault, 1990: 140).[34] This applies to the checkpoints at neighbourhood entrances and the requirement for Palestinians to obtain permits for hospital appointments in Jerusalem.[35] In entering these spaces and being subject to these exclusionary structures and practices, Palestinians become 'bare life' (Agamben, 1998: 8)[36] that can be violently targeted. Israel seeks 'the generalized instrumentalization of human existence and the material destruction of human bodies and populations' (Mbembe, 2003: 14)[37] through the initiation and application of a necropolitics that creates 'death-worlds' (Mbembe, 2003: 14).

H2 Palestinians endure frequent acts of settler terrorism[38] and extrajudicial killings by the Israeli army.[39] In Hebron, settlers are in control, to the point where they feel they can order Israeli soldiers to kill Palestinians. A captain of the Israeli army who served in Hebron in 2010 confirms that '[t]here's no doubt that [the Israeli army] worked for the settlers', [and adds] [s]ettler representatives arrived at the briefings. There are civilian security coordinators (settlers in charge of the security of the settlement, appointed by the Ministry of Defense), but there's also someone who coordinates it, a civilian (Breaking the Silence, 2017: 38).[40]

One Israeli sergeant and member of 'Breaking the Silence',[41] who served in the territories in 2017, recalls that '[w]e really hated the children of the [settler] families in the Red House who shouted at us, "How come you're not killing the Palestinians passing by there?" They saw us letting Palestinians pass by: "Why do you let him pass? Kill him"' (Breaking the Silence, 2018: 32).[42] Fawaz Abu Aiysheh, who has recently left Tel Rumeida, observes the settlers are a 'mafia' 'who are more vicious and brutal because there are no consequences to their actions'.[43] It is no surprise that Israel does not want the world to see what goes on here – in January 2019, it expelled the Temporary International Presence in Hebron (TIPH) that had previously documented and recorded Israeli violations and provided a degree of protection to Palestinians.

Settlers, including the notorious Anat Cohen, whose violent assaults on Palestinians[44] and international activists have turned her into something of a celebrity,[45] carry out their violent provocations in the knowledge and expectation they will be protected by Israeli soldiers.[46] After settlers seized a Tel Rumeida house in 2001, it took almost twenty years for an Israeli court to rule they should be evicted. In response, Peace Now observed that this was, in addition to the 'cruelty, deceit and theft of settlers', also attributable to a 'lack of government accountability'. It observed the government did not just fail to enforce the law but also helped the settlers to steal the house and terrorize their Palestinian neighbours.[47]

Settler attacks occur more frequently in Hebron and the surrounding area than anywhere else in the West Bank. In a B'Tselem video, one Tel Rumeida observes that '[i]f I file[d] a complaint about every assault, I'd have no time to go work'.[48] Yesh Din[49] observes that '[c]ompared to overall figures for the West Bank, the rate of violent incidence in the city is particularly high: While violence accounts for 35 percent of the incidents documented by Yesh Din in the West Bank as a whole, 62 percent of the incidents documented in Hebron were violent offenses' (2018).[50]

Israeli restrictions in H2 turn everyday tasks into a time-consuming ordeal. Ayat Hamdan explains how one of her interviewees, who has asthma, was prevented from receiving essential materials by Israeli soldiers, despite receiving Rehabilitation Committee approval.[51]

Hamdan observes '[t]he furnishing of homes can also take a long time. Moving each individual piece of furniture through military checkpoints is a laborious undertaking'. One of her interviewees took six months to move all of her furniture into her home (2020: 121).[52]

In the Tel Rumeida neighbourhood, which lies to the west of the Old City, Israel prevents non-residents from entering and also forbids residents from driving cars, which gravely impacts those with special needs (these movement restrictions also apply in H1 areas). Ambulances are not allowed to enter certain areas and experience delays when seeking to reach patients. Taysir Abu 'Ayeshe tried to walk his pregnant wife to the hospital after she began bleeding at 2 am. However, by the time they reached the hospital, she had lost the baby.[53] Nour,[54] a former resident of Tel Rumeida, told me about her experience of living there:

> [T]he checkpoint was down the street. I witnessed 8 Palestinians killed by Israeli soldiers, Israeli settlers encourage them to kill. It really affected me and my family . . . my children used to wake up at night screaming.[. . .] we had a factory near the settlement in the old city, we had 40 workers. Settlers' attacks and intimidations led many to leave. The attacks were serious, we were near death, by the time of the second intifada we were only three family members remained to work at the factory.

Nour further explains,

> By the time of the second intifada we were only three family members remained to work at the factory. As the second intifada started, we

received an Israeli military order of closure. Setters' attacks protected by Israeli soldiers. Once Anat Cohen attacked my wife and hit her. I went to police station to complain. While waiting outside, Anat walked in, after a while and when she left, they called me. When I explained what happened, they told me that I am under investigation due to a complaint from Anat and had to go to court and if failed to show up, will pay a high fine. I had to solicit a lawyer, then they dismissed the case. This is a message for us not to think of complaining when attacked by settlers.

Residents unsurprisingly do not want to remain here. Nour told me: 'There are families who leave and others move in. Families with children and teenagers, usually move out. Older families without children move in because of cheap rents there.' Of the 3,369 housing units here, a third are empty because of settler attacks. It is possible to rent houses for a low price (B'Tselem, 2019: 22–3).[55] Nour adds it is no surprise that parents outside do not want their daughters to get married there, as 'they don't want their daughters to be killed'.[56]

One of Hamdan's interviewees observes:

We suffer from an invisible problem, which is the difficulty of marrying our daughters under these circumstances. Young men who propose marriage to women who do not live in this area are usually rejected. In the long run this is a very serious issue for the new generation because they are forced to leave their homes and the family's house in order to marry and start a family. When many children reached the age of marriage, they had to leave the area. (2020: 122)[57]

And it is difficult enough to get permission to live there (and also in Hebron more generally) in the first place. Badil observes:

Denial of residency in Hebron takes the form of denying Palestinians the right to choose and maintain their residency in certain neighborhoods. . . . Retaining residency in closed military zones is dependent on continuous residence within its premises, as the right to residency is lost as soon as one relocates outside of the designated zone. As a result, families face many difficulties when they relocate for safety, security, or movement issues but still want to look after the home they were forced to vacate. (2016a: 36)[58]

In these closed or restricted areas, Palestinian movement is restricted and regulated by Israeli checkpoints. Palestinians in the Old City are attacked every day (both verbally and physically) by Israeli settlers, and have even been forced to install metal wire mesh on their windows to protect themselves from settlers throwing objects at their homes (2016b: 31).[59] Israeli soldiers also impose collective punishments, including closures (B'Tselem, 2015).[60] Negative economic, education and health-related (especially psychological) impacts are experienced every day.[61] In this 'coercive environment', Palestinians face 'forcible transfer' (Badil, 2016)[62] and are subject to policies of erasure enacted through army-settler cooperation (Halper, 2021; Wolfe, 2006).[63] Qurei, the chief Palestinian negotiator in the Oslo Accords, who was not part of the Hebron negotiations, observes that 'Israel made a fatal mistake for not withdrawing the Israeli settlers from Hebron and so did the Palestinian leadership [by] not insisting on [this]' (2005: 308).[64]

In the South Hebron Hills, which are part of Area C, around 4,000 Palestinians live with the perpetual threat of displacement. They have no access to water or electricity, are subject to repeated and extensive Israeli violence,[65] and are forbidden from building unless they obtain construction permits from Israel.[66] The Hills are part of the Masafer Yatta area, which include about 30 villages that contain 4,000 Palestinian farmers and shepherds. In Area 918, a designated firing zone, around twelve communities mostly live in caves and work in agriculture (mostly sheep herding). The residents are surrounded by four main settlements (Ma'on, Susiya, Beit Yattir and Karmel) and ten outposts. Here, as elsewhere in Area C, Israel effectively bans any construction or installation of basic services.[67] Israel destroys donor-funded alternative energy sources, such as solar panels, by drawing on settler information obtained through various means, including the flying of surveillance drones.[68] When donors such as Belgium (and other EU Member States) seek compensation, Israel rejects the claims, and cites the illegality of constructing in firing zones in 'justification'.[69]

The pandemic in Hebron

In July 2020, Hebron became a pandemic epicentre, accounting for 70 per cent of West Bank cases.[70] This was attributable to a number of factors, including Israel's demolition of a coronavirus quarantine centre,[71] as part of a targeting of health clinics across the West Bank in the pandemic[72] and the H1/H2 arrangement, which has also hindered Palestinian law enforcement efforts.[73]

Nour Abu Aisha, a merchant who used to live in the Old City and Tel Rumeida and who currently lives in H2, claims that the Palestinian police initially tried to introduce preventative and protective measures in H1 but were obstructed by the Israelis. He claims that Israel used Covid-19 as a pretext to impose restrictions on Palestinians – he notes, for example, that it closed the Ibrahami mosque for Palestinian prayers but allowed Jews to enter.[74]

Dr Hazem Alshhab told me, 'In H2 PA could provide services. [This included] personal efforts and [cooperation with] volunteers and international organisations. In Area C, these efforts established mobile clinics.' [And he added]

> 'At the beginning of the outbreak of the virus, [the] PA declared [a] state of emergency and imposed closure. However, PA has no power over large area of the West Bank. The division of the land has a great impact on ability to combat the virus. PA has no control over H2 and cannot impose law there. This contributed to the spread of the virus.'[75]

He observes that Israel did not take measures and notes that it was only Palestinians who work in the settlements that were tested and later vaccinated. He adds that Israel will only intervene if there is an attack on settlers and will do nothing to address internal Palestinian fighting.[76]

Another interviewee further explained the impact of division on PA measures,

> At the outbreak of the virus and early on, people complied with measures and lockdown. Dora is inside the municipality boundary. The lockdown was managed by local councils…people closed entrances to

villages, although area C, Israeli army didn't object. If they wanted to arrest someone, they remove barrels and enter. Most western villages of Hebron are area C and the roads to settlements.[77]

PA also coordinates with Israel to enter the off-limit areas. For example, a few days following the vaccination scandal, Palestinian security forces killed Nizar Banat, an activist, critical of PA arrested Banat several times previously and he was subject to harassments and intimidated actions. This time and in June 24 security forces broke into the house of his family in H2 area at dawn and arrested Banat violently. Banat was brutally beaten with rods and batons, which led to his death.[78] One of the interviewees, whom I interviewed the same day Banat was killed, explained to me how role of PA in H2 is limited to intelligence activities in cooperation with Israel,

> Today PA killed Nizar Banat, he was staying in H2 Area with his relatives to avoid arrest. Israel bans PA security forces from entering the area. PA never chased people who commit criminal acts and take refuge in H2. To arrest Nizar Banat, PA coordinated with Israel, this part of the security coordination.[79]

Areas beyond PA reach became a refuge for outlaws and avoiding prosecution.[80] As mentioned earlier, Israel banned Palestinian security forces to operate in H2 to enforce corona measures.

The politicization of the Covid-19 response was also highlighted as an important factor by interviewees, and to this extent Fatah's monopolization of the emergency committees excluded Palestinian civil society[81] and negatively impacted wider public opinion. It also failed to meet public health requirements – one Tel Rumeida resident told me that a Fatah initiative provided masks, but not for everyone.[82] Fawaz Abu Aisheh, in referring to the PA's corruption, similarly highlights its limited and selective implementation of public health measures. Fatah activities were protected by security forces, while others were banned.[83] Politicization also refers to the privileging of specific cities and power bases during the pandemic. Ashhab, for instance, criticizes the Minister of Health for not paying attention to Hebron at the peak of the pandemic. He explains that while 'Hebron is one third of [the] West Bank, [the] Minister of Health visited only 2 or 3 time[s]. [The] PA['s] main focus is Ramallah, it is about show off, photos and media.'[84] Fuad al-Amour, an activist and coordinator of the Protection and Sumud Committee, claimed that the PA's service provision in the South Hebron Hills also left much to be desired. He observed that the

> PA provided some safety equipment, like masks and sanitisers, but only sporadic[ally] and through companies. They come to distribute parcels, take pictures and never show up again. Also, Area C in south Hebron Hills is underdeveloped and depends on Yatta city. When PA imposed lockdown, we were unable to purchase essentials and basic materials, PA did provide any alternatives. Israeli doesn't allow PA to operate in Area C. When Palestinian ministry of health tried to provide coronavirus testing tent, Israel removed it within three days and confiscated material. Even International donors can only provide some safety material, but Israel doesn't allow them to build centers.[85]

Politicization was also linked to public fears about the vaccine. One interviewee told me: 'It is fear not lack of awareness, due to the news about the expired vaccine, and conflicting news. People are afraid of vaccine, no confidence, people believe that [the] vaccine will lead to death.'[86] Another interviewee told me she doesn't trust Palestinian hospitals. She said: '[W]e feel we are used as trials, people have no confidence. My son and myself had corona, but did not go to the hospital, we know from the symptoms, we lost taste and smell senses. I treated myself and my son, with antibiotics and painkillers.'[87] Fuad al-Amour echoed this, noting '[n]ow after the scandal of the vaccine, there is vaccine hesitancy. For us corona is not a priority for us, people hardly mention it. People are facing eviction and settler attacks.'[88] However, another interviewee noted vaccination is a requirement for travel, which will incentivize Palestinians to get vaccinated and take the 'expensive' Covid-19 test.[89]

Fatah's monopolization of the emergency committees and the resulting exclusion of civil society also helps to explain the inefficiencies of the pandemic response in Palestine.[90] This has not just weakened the committees but has also strengthened (the already strong) popular mistrust of the political authorities.

The PA imposed a lockdown in response to the escalating situation. However, Palestinians who worked in Israel did not have the option of not working and so continued to travel to Israel to work, jeopardizing their own health and the health of those around them. Israel, meanwhile, continued to issue work permits and even turned a blind eye to Palestinians entering Israel through holes in the wall.[91] Hisham Sharabati[92] claims this was deliberate and was intended to convey the clear message that Israel was the ultimate political authority in the territory. The Palestine New Federation of Trade Unions observed the pandemic made it clear that capitalism and colonialism spoke a common language of 'discrimination, exploitation and racism', and claimed that the line that differentiates 'lives that matter' from 'those that don't matter' was drawn more clearly 'than ever before'.[93] Samour echoes this by presenting the decisions of Palestinian workers as a consequence of a land dispossession that left them with no option but to seek employment in the Israeli labour market (2020: 58).[94] He accordingly speaks of a 'necroeconomy' that exposes workers to death (2020: 56)[95] and clarifies

> Workers' calculus to work under such conditions is not only determined by the lack of a safety buffer in the form of health, unemployment, or paid leave insurance, but more fundamentally, by the cruel compulsion of capitalism that leaves them with no choice but to work to live at the risk of exposure to death. (2020: 56)[96]

Fawaz Abu Aisheh claims that H1 residents originally observed lockdown measures but were forced to re-evaluate when they realized it 'meant no work and no income'. Furthermore, the PA, in citing Israel's decision to withhold tax revenues after the PA opposed its annexation plan,[97] was not in a position to provide full compensation and could only pay half of salaries.[98] Manal, a single mother from Tel Rumeida, claims '[t]he PA has no mercy and people know that'. She explains, 'lockdown affected us badly. Now with omicron variant, PA takes no action. PA has to compensate us if we have shut down, I am a single mother because my husband is martyr, he died from teargas in 2015. As a single mother I have to feed my kids'.[99]

Necropolitics also applies in another sense, namely to Israel's land-focused colonial activities. This is a necropolitical power exerted by the Israeli army and settlers (Mbembe, 2003: 29).[100] Indeed, Israeli soldiers and settlers do not just impede efforts to prevent the spread of the virus but also appear to do their best to actively encourage it. Nour Abu Aisha told me that 'Israeli settlers and soldiers, at the peak of virus, used to spit on Palestinians houses and cars. They used to touch the handles of doors of Palestinians to spread the virus in Tel Rumeida and old city. No measures were taken during arrests, we heard in Israeli news there are positive cases among soldiers'.[101]

Fawaz Abu Aisheh observes that Israel used fines for vindictive and not public health reasons, and claims that 'soldiers and settlers [who were in some cases infected] tried to spread the virus by spitting on peoples' houses, coughing and touching their door handles'.[102] Another resident confirms that Israeli settlers spat on Palestinian residents and their cars. In observing that Israel did initially fine those who refused to wear masks, they noted that Israeli military operations did not comply with social distancing requirements.[103] Fuad al-Amour referred to an incident in the South Hills of Hebron, where masked and socially distanced settlers deliberately started a fire, with the apparent intention of forcing Palestinians to mix and encouraging virus spread.[104] The likelihood of such provocations was further increased by the decline in international activism during the pandemic. However, as Fuad al-Amour notes, the Israeli army was at least less likely to use tear gas when Israeli activists were present.[105]

Hazem Ashhab observes cases had begun to decline by summer 2021 and, in support of this claim, notes there were no Covid-19 patients in his hospital. He cites both travel restrictions and closures, which he claims prevented new variants from developing.[106] Even during the pandemic, economic considerations predominated in residents' considerations, and it appears even more likely that this will be the case now. Similarly, the colonization of Palestinian land and settler violence did not go away during the pandemic and continued to impose themselves on residents.[107] Covid-19 also affected these economic pressures – one interviewee notes it, in combination with drought and water shortages, caused the price of animal feed to double. They note this will force rural residents to move to cities, which will in turn strengthen Israel's grip on the oPt.[108]

Conclusion

In the bloody and chaotic aftermath of Barack Goldstein's notorious massacre, Hebron has always been where the apartheid character of Israel's colonization has been most clearly displayed. The 'security' measures introduced by Israel in the aftermath of the massacre, and most notably the Hebron Protocol, grossly infringe on hundreds of thousands of Hebron residents for the benefit of a few hundred Israeli settlers. Some lives are clearly worth more than others, and some are condemned to die so others may live. This was the reality before the pandemic, and will also be the reality after it. Similarly, while colonialism may have impacted aspects of the pandemic, and the pandemic may have impacted particular colonial arrangements, the essential character of colonialism persisted.

The H1/H2 administrative divide impacts on all aspects of life in the city, and so it was no surprise that interviewees most frequently cited it as the key factor that contributed to virus spread in the early stages of the pandemic, and stressed its importance in Hebron emerging as the virus epicentre of the West Bank and, at one point, accounting for more than two-thirds of total recorded cases. However, this is to assume that the PA response in the city would have been more effective if it had been permitted to operate in H2 – however, as previous chapters have highlighted the inefficiencies and shortcomings in the PA's pandemic response, this assertion appears to be, at best, open to question. In other words, there are few, if any grounds, for assuming that the PA's response would have been any more effective if this obstacle had not existed or been removed.

While interviewees sometimes disagreed on the extent of the public health measures that were introduced (some said there were none, whereas others pointed to limited preventative measures), there was nonetheless a general consensus that the response was inadequate and that the PA failed to sufficiently address the challenge. This reflects the impact of the fragmentation of Hebron and the limited spaces available for Palestinians to operate. This was perhaps most obvious in the failure to fully compensate workers, with the result that they were frequently forced to prioritize economic survival over their own health and the health and well-being of their families and the wider community. Accordingly, even during spikes in the pandemic, residents of Hebron did not regard it as their foremost priority.

This raises the question of what role the PA should have actually played in leading the pandemic response. Low levels of public popularity and support raise the question of if it would have been better for an independent authority to provide guidance and support – the obvious reference point here is the Palestinian leadership of the First *Intifada* who were able to promote popular mobilization and direct collective energies towards clearly defined goals. In this respect, I found it instructive to refer to one of my previous publications, which examined the role of the Palestinian leadership in the First *Intifada*. I specifically recalled how activists told me how the leadership had the trust of the people and played an effective role in mobilizing the masses to resist the occupation. Ala Alazzeh observes that '[a]mong activists today, there is a strong anxiety about the lack of popular participation and an attendant nostalgia for and desire to reproduce the ethos of the First *Intifada*' (2015: 264).[109]

The PA is clearly not able to perform this role or assume this responsibility. Interviewees also raised concerns about the politicization of the pandemic response and the extent to which the PA sought to manipulate it for its own political advantage and purposes. This linked into separate concerns about the independence of health authorities, the dispersal of health resources and persistent fears about the safety of the vaccine that were further exacerbated, and exemplified, by the notorious vaccine scandal which aside from illustrating the PA's political shortcomings also underlined the neo-colonial terms on which Palestinians, and others across the world, are expected to receive health provision.

It is perhaps surprising to observe that Israel did not just fail to coordinate with the PA in responding to the pandemic, but actually sought to undermine it, including by acting in a manner that could potentially undermine its own public health measures. The 'necroeconomy' based on the exploitation of human suffering and disadvantage therefore persisted, despite the fact that permitting potentially infected Palestinians to travel to Israel potentially jeopardized the health and well-being of Israelis. It is considerably less surprising that within Hebron itself, Israeli soldiers and settlers deliberately – including by spitting on door handles and disrupting extremely limited preventative measures in place – sought to encourage virus spread among residents. This clearly reiterated and underlined the extent of Israel's contempt for Palestinian lives.

Existence as non-existence
The pandemic in Kufr ʿAqab

Introduction

This chapter examines how Israel's efforts to combat the pandemic in Jerusalem have systematically discriminated against the 350,000 Palestinians who live in East Jerusalem alongside more than 200,000 Israeli settlers.[1] It provides a case study of Kufr ʿAqab that examines the different measures Israel has used to hinder Palestinians, a number of which predate the pandemic.

This discrimination is confirmed by a recent Human Rights Watch report, which observes that '[a]cross [the occupied Palestinian territories and Israel] and in most aspects of life, Israeli authorities methodically privilege Jewish Israelis and discriminate against Palestinians'.[2] Quiet deportation is just one example of this. It has previously been observed that it is a direct continuation of Israel's overall policy in East Jerusalem since 1967 that is implemented with the aim of preserving a permanent majority of Jews in the city and ensuring that Israel's 'sovereignty' in East Jerusalem cannot be challenged (HaMoked and B'Tselem, 1997: 41).[3]

This demands action across a range of spheres. Israel has taken various actions with the aim of forcing Palestinian Jerusalemites to leave, including by deliberately impeding development, demolishing homes, expropriating land, restricting (Palestinian) access to land and passing laws that revoke (Palestinian) residency[4]. Israel considers Jerusalem to be its united capital and has repeatedly and vehemently rejected the proposition it should be divided and shared with Palestinians.

Land confiscation and settlement activity (in, but particularly around, the city) are clearly intended to alter the city's demographic balance. De facto annexation (Bishara, 2001: 84–95)[5] is enabled and advanced by a general approach of 'constructive ambiguity' that deliberately blurs and conceals the occupier's intentions and practices. Eyal Weizman invokes it when he refers to an arrangement in which the fragmentation of land and frontiers are not 'rigid' but 'elastic, and in constant transformation' (2007: 6).[6] He further clarifies:

> The linear border, a cartographic imaginary inherited from the military and political spatiality of the nation state has splintered into a multitude of temporary, transportable, deployable and removable border-synonyms – 'separation walls', 'barriers', 'blockades', 'closures', 'road blocks', 'checkpoints', 'sterile areas', 'special security zones', 'closed military areas' and 'killing zones' – that shrink and expand the territory at will. (2007: 6)[7]

The Palestinian narrative in Jerusalem is also targeted by Israeli attacks. The Israeli Ministry of Education previously censored Palestinian textbooks and imposed changes, including replacing the Palestinian logo with the Jerusalem municipality logo. It also deleted the Palestinian flag, along with all sections related to Palestinian history or the *Nakba*. In some cases, no effort was made to conceal this and the deleted pages were left blank.[8] Schools were not allowed to purchase their textbooks from any source other than the municipality and if they tried to do this, they risked losing funding and access to resources.[9] These measures of control and surveillance were complemented by pre-established counterparts.[10]

Ziad al Shamali, the head of the parents' committee union, explained that although Palestinian education has been targeted for more than a decade, Israel's efforts have intensified over the last three years. He refers to 'an Israelisation of Palestinian education'.[11] This recalls Grande's observation that 'Indian education was never simply about the desire to "civilize" or even deculturalize a people'; instead, she suggests it was always 'designed to colonize Indian minds as a means of gaining access to Indian labor, land, and resources' (2015: 23).[12]

Israel also restricts Palestinian urban development and this is shown, for example, by the conditions that it imposes on town planning schemes, which make it expensive and time-consuming to seek municipal approval for permits. As a result, many Palestinian Jerusalemites have built without permits, despite the risk of demolition and of their homes being added to the list of around 803 houses destroyed in the period 2004–18.[13] Israel's policy of constructing national parks in East Jerusalem also enables it to increase the Jewish presence, impede Palestinian development/Palestinian residents and link the Old City to the E1 settlement.[14]

And the 'Centre of Life Law' requires Palestinians to maintain a permanent presence in the city – those who leave, including those who leave the West Bank for seven years or become a citizen of another country, could have their residency revoked (HaMoKed & B'Tselem, 1997: 10).[15] In 1995, the policy was extended to the rest of the West Bank,[16] meaning that Jerusalemites who live in Ramallah, for example, risk having their residency revoked. In the period after 1967, more than 14,500 Palestinians have been stripped of residency.[17]

This chapter demonstrates how the division of Palestinians into different spaces is part of a colonial tactic that seeks to create 'compartments' (Fanon, 1963: 37).[18] Joronen, in developing this concept, observes how it creates 'precarious zones' where the colonized is subject to different forms of violence on a daily basis (2019: 840).[19] One of the key developments in this regard was Israel's 1992 introduction of a permit system that separated Jerusalem from the rest of the West Bank.

In this chapter, I will examine how Israel uses colonial tactics (Veracini, 2010)[20] to control Kufr 'Aqab's residents by deliberately curtailing their links to Jerusalem city and forcing them to look for alternatives. Tanous notes:

> Violent bureaucratic practices, such as revocation of residency statuses and the prevention of family reunification laws, add layers

of exhaustion to the lives of Palestinian Jerusalemites. On top of their daily obstacles, they have to continuously prove to the occupier that they actually have a right to live in their city; that they are not infiltrators or illegal residents.[21]

This chapter will focus in particular on 'centre of life' and family unification policies, which have a huge impact on residents' lives. Indeed, many residents live here to meet the 'centre of life' requirements. This is why they speak of it as a 'functional' space and directly contrast it with a traditional Palestinian society, where neighbours and surrounding communities are familiar and known (Hammoudeh, Hamayel and Welchman, 2016: 47).[22]

In order to understand the challenges that residents of Kufr 'Aqab face in the pandemic, I will refer to broader Israeli colonial policies that seek to 'eliminate' the Palestinian presence in the city. The imposed necropolitical reality produces the 'living dead', 'pain' (Mbembe, 2003: 39)[23] and 'bare life' (1998: 81–6).[24] Here, as in the Gaza Strip, residents are forced to continually respond and react to a perpetual 'state of exception' (Abujidi, 2009: 272).[25]

Hammoudeh observes that 'many residents described community unease and fear in building social relations', and adds that '[t]hese feelings generated an unwillingness to form neighborly bonds, with mistrust permeating communities' (2016: 46). This affected my own work, as I struggled to find interviewees – acquaintances could not refer me to other residents or even their own neighbours because they have almost no social relations with them.

Most interviewees preferred to remain anonymous in order to guard against the possibility that the Israeli government might vindictively retaliate by revoking the residency applications of spouses and children. I accordingly removed any additional details that could reveal their identities. Although for purposes of clarity, I distinguish between Palestinians with 'permanent residency' (holders of a Jerusalem ID) and those without (holders of West Bank ID), this distinction has no basis in international law, which regards East Jerusalem as part of the West Bank.

Historical background

On 19 February 1947, Ernest Bevin, the British foreign secretary, announced he would hand over the Palestine problem to the United Nations. In the following May, a meeting of the General Assembly appointed a United Nations Special Commission (UNSCOP) for Palestine and asked it to provide recommendations. It eventually proposed that Palestine should be partitioned into Jewish and Arab states and that Jerusalem should be placed under international jurisdiction. One day after the UN vote, Menachem Begin, the Irgun commander who later became Israel's prime minister, said: 'The partition of Palestine is illegal. It will never be recognized. . . . Jerusalem was and will forever be our capital. Eretz Israel will be restored to the people of Israel. All of it. And for ever' (Shlaim, 2000: 28).[26]

The Haganah expelled Palestinians from the western part of the city (in violation of international law), and Jordan occupied the eastern half. In 1950, the Knesset passed a law that proclaimed Jerusalem to be Israel's capital, and the government then began to move buildings to the city. Thirty years later, a Basic Law amendment declared the city to be the country's 'united capital'.

Judaization of the city began almost immediately after the end of the 1967 Six-Day War. The Absentee Property Law (1950), which was originally used to seize Palestinian property after the 1948 war, was extended to the city. Israel annexed East Jerusalem, bestowed the 'permanent resident' status on its 230,000 Palestinian residents and expanded the city's municipal borders with the aim of shifting the demographic balance in favour of Israeli Jews. This established a clear distinction between the city's Palestinian residents and their oPt counterparts. Palestinian Jerusalemites do not require a permit to enter or work in Israel and are permitted to vote, albeit only in local elections that are generally boycotted in any case. While this residency can be inherited, the family reunification process is, as we will see, drawn out and prolonged. These rights, along with the rights of tourists and other non-citizens, are regulated by the entry into Israel Law and associated regulations (Jeffries, 2012: 97).[27]

After the 1967 War, Israel prevented Palestinian residents of Jerusalem who were absent or who had fled or were expelled from returning. It destroyed the Old City's Maghribi Quarter, which was built in 1320, and confiscated about 600 dunams of Old City land to build the Jewish Quarter while invoking a dubious 'public use' pretext in justification. These actions were consistent with the Allon Plan's proposed expropriation and annexation of Palestinian land (Raz, 2012: 244–7).[28] Israel expanded the city's municipal boundaries while expropriating more than a third of it and also built settlements. This was deliberately intended to incorporate the city's Jewish population and exclude Palestinians, whose villages and neighbourhoods were divided as a result.

The sensitivities that surround the city were clearly shown in the 1978 peace negotiations between Egypt and Israel, and were directly acknowledged by Jimmy Carter, the then US president, in a formal communication to Anwar Sadat, the then Egyptian president.[29] The city was excluded from the final agreement. The Oslo Accords also refused to directly address Jerusalem and deferred it to a later stage of negotiations. In the pre-Oslo negotiations, Uri Savir, Israel's chief negotiator, made it clear to his Palestinian counterparts that his government viewed this as a precondition for continued negotiations (1998: 15).[30] On 2 June 1996, after his victory in the preceding election, Benjamin Netanyahu clearly pre-empted 'final status' negotiations when he said: 'We will keep Jerusalem united under Israeli sovereignty. I declare this here tonight in Jerusalem, the eternal capital of the Jewish people which will never be divided.'[31]

Between May 1996 and 1999, Netanyahu took unilateral actions, including opening a tunnel close to Al-Aqsa mosque/Al-Haram al-Sharif and also allowed settlers to seize Jabal Abu Ghunim in East Jerusalem and start building a new housing project. Rising Palestinian anger sparked the 'tunnel uprising', when clashes between Palestinians (including police) and the Israeli army left sixty-one Palestinians and fifteen Israelis dead. Palestinian suicide bombers also struck Israel on 30 July and 4 September 1997.

The 2000 Camp David negotiations did not challenge Israel's control over the city but instead proposed to further cement the instruments and mechanisms it had put in place in East Jerusalem, including the construction of illegal settlements on confiscated land, home demolitions, the confiscation of ID cards and the imposition of closures that economically choked the city and cut it off from the rest of the West Bank (Bishara, 2001: 90).[32]

As the negotiations stalled, the city once again moved to the foreground. On 28 September 2001, Ariel Sharon, the Likud leader, visited the city's Haram al-Sharif and lit the fuse that sparked the Second/Al-Aqsa *Intifada*. Israel responded by imposing closures, land confiscations and checkpoints on Palestinians (OCHA, 2008).[33] The mosque has more recently emerged as a flashpoint after a proposed law that would allow metal detectors to be placed at the entrance was dropped in response to US pressure and Palestinian protests.[34]

In 2002, Israel began to construct a wall, with the aim of effectively annexing 'bordering' areas of the Palestinian West Bank. Elia Zureik explains:

> The wall itself has resulted in the expropriation of 10 per cent of Palestinian lands. Bearing in mind that the West Bank and Gaza constituted 28 per cent of the area of Mandate Palestine, land expropriation for roads, the wall, and above all new settlements, is expected to reduce the size of the Palestinian enclaves to no more that 45 per cent of the area of the West Bank, which is almost 15 per cent of the area of historical Palestine. (2016: 99)[35]

The wall, whose construction destroyed houses and uprooted trees, also separates families and seals Jerusalem off from the rest of the West Bank (OCHA, 2011).[36] In 2004, the International Court of Justice (ICJ) declared the wall was illegal. However, Israel persists in viewing it as a border and has introduced a permit system for Palestinians.

After the terrorist attacks of 11 September 2001 in the United States, the rhetoric of the 'War on Terror' enabled Israel to expand and strengthen its control over Palestinians (Berda, 2017).[37] In 2003, following the outbreak of the Second *Intifada*, the Knesset passed a law that temporarily halted all reunification applications. This law remains in force at the time of writing, meaning that residency continues to be refused to Palestinians (with PA ID) who are married to Israeli citizens or with Jerusalem ID. They are not currently even allowed to enter the city.[38]

In any case, Israel had already imposed electoral requirements that restricted the ability of Palestinian Jerusalemites to stand for election. Savir observes that '[e]ach Palestinian candidate living in Jerusalem would be required to have a second, binding address outside the city, making it possible for Israel to claim that no Palestinian Jerusalemite was standing for election' (Savir, 1998: 221).[39] In 2021, it went further and banned Palestinian Jerusalemites from voting in the scheduled Palestinian legislative elections, leading Abbas to postpone them in protest.[40]

In 2018, the Knesset amended the law to allow the interior minister to revoke Palestinian residency in the event of a 'breach of allegiance to the State of Israel'.[41] In response, various organizations[42] issued a critical joint statement. They observe:

> This law is unconstitutional and is intended to result in the illegal expulsion of Palestinians from Jerusalem, the city of their birth. Even though the revocation of residency entails a severe violation of basic rights – including the right to family, the right to free movement, and the right to freedom of employment – members of the Knesset nevertheless chose to grant the interior minister the authority to do as he wishes. East Jerusalem is occupied territory, and its Palestinian residents are a protected population under international humanitarian law. It is therefore forbidden to impose upon them an obligation of loyalty to Israel, let alone revoke their permanent residency status for 'breach of loyalty', essentially resulting in their expulsion from the city.[43]

The Knesset did not extend the law in July 2021, which was perhaps surprising given that Yair Lapid, the country's foreign minister, candidly acknowledged its intention and purpose when he said: '[There's] no need to hide from the purpose of the [citizenship] law, it's one of the tools meant to secure a Jewish majority in Israel. Israel is the nation-state of the Jewish people, and our goal is that it will have a Jewish majority.'[44] In fact, the Ministry of Interior continued to revoke the status of Palestinians in Jerusalem based on 'breach of loyalty' to present time.[45]

On 6 December 2017, Trump recognized Jerusalem as the capital of Israel, before moving the US embassy from Tel Aviv to the city on 16 May of the following year. And on 30 June 2019, David Friedman, the US ambassador to Israel, joined Israeli settlers at the inauguration of a tunnel opening that led to Al-Aqsa Mosque.[46]

In various areas of the Old City, such as Abu Dis, Ras al-'Amud, Sheikh Jarrah and Silwan, Israeli settlers are now, with the support of the Israeli authorities, seeking to evict Palestinians from their homes and replace them. In doing so, they invoke a 1970 law that allows Israelis to reclaim property in East Jerusalem. Palestinians resisting in Sheikh Jarrah view the contemporary evictions as the latest story in a history of dispossession that extends back to the *Nakba*.

An introduction to Kufr 'Aqab

Kufr 'Aqab is based in the north-east of Jerusalem and is bordered by Ramallah Governorate to the East and Qalandiya Camp to the South. It has been transformed in the period since 1967: 30 per cent of the village is a neighbourhood of the municipality of Jerusalem and the remainder is part of Area C. It is the best location in the Jerusalem municipality for couples with Jerusalem and West Bank IDs, and it is where many Palestinians wait for their residency applications to be completed. Nonetheless, in the words of one interviewee, they are only here because they have 'no other choice'.[47] Hammoudeh, Hamayel and Welchman observe:

> [R]elocation to Kufr 'Aqab has helped Israel's policies of displacement succeed. These policies have forced residents to constantly have to

'prove their existence', which they must substantiate with meticulous documentation attesting to a connection with Jerusalem as well as intrusive investigations that cause community disintegration and negatively impact sense of belonging, and therefore wellbeing. (2016: 47)[48]

Kufr 'Aqab is part of Israel's policies in East Jerusalem, which include evicting Palestinians from Shiekh Jarrah, and is a continuation of Israel's concern with altering the 'demographic balance' in the city – as Khalil Tofakji, a Palestinian expert and cartographer, observes, this has been an established priority for Israel since 1967 (2000: 54).[49] And it should therefore be understood in the lineage of plans, such as those announced in 1990 by Ariel Sharon who, in his role as minister of housing construction, proposed the construction of settlement blocs in the middle of Palestinian neighbourhoods in the city, with the aim of encircling, fragmenting and dispersing Palestinian residents.[50]

Kufr 'Aqab is located beyond the wall and is cut off from Jerusalem, but it remains open and accessible to Ramallah and other Area A residents. The Separation/Apartheid Wall cut off 140,000 Palestinian Jerusalemites who lived within the city's municipal boundaries in areas such as Shu'fat Refugee Camp and Kafr 'Aqab, and directly impacted their lives by fragmentating land (Ophir and Hanafi, 2009).[51] Jerusalemites, who live 'beyond the wall', are particularly impacted by Israeli building permit restrictions, spousal reunification policies (Ir Amim, n.d.)[52] and checkpoints that make it difficult to access health and medical services and treatments in Jerusalem. Couples from Kufr 'Aqab with different IDs are treated differently when they cross checkpoints. One interviewee spoke of her experiences travelling with her two children:

> When I travelled to Jordan, my two children, 2 and 6, with Jerusalem ID were taken from me by Israeli soldier, with a gun, to cross from a different side than the one I should use as a WB ID'. One time, I was trying to cross the checkpoint to Jerusalem with my children, the soldier told me that they are not allowed cross without the presence

of their father, who holds the Jerusalem ID. The soldier told me that the children are registered with their father and his responsibility. I started to scream at the soldiers saying 'they are with me because I am their mother'. They held me for some time and did not cross. If I cross the checkpoint with them alone, soldiers need to see their birth certificate.[53]

Kufr 'Aqab is part of Israel's designs for the wider West Bank, which include the construction of settlements in anticipation of eventual annexation. Israel is currently building a bypass ring ('The American Road'), with the aim of linking northern and southern settlements. Land confiscation and demolition will occur in various areas, including Kufr 'Aqab, and Jerusalem will eventually be disconnected from the rest of the West Bank.[54]

Munir Zughayer[55] refers, for example, to Israel's proposal to create a local council for Kufr 'Aqab, which he presents as part of Israel's plan for a 'Greater Jerusalem' that will minimize the number of Palestinians in the city (see ACRI, 2017).[56] He notes it was rejected by local residents who unanimously believed services should be provided by Jerusalem Municipality.[57] Jamal Juma, however, claims that 'Israel has no definitive plan for Kufr 'Aqab' and suggests that the proposal is a way of 'testing the water' in preparation for residents being incorporated into PA administration. He suggests it was put forward because of Israel's fear that Palestinians will participate in municipality elections that they currently boycott.[58]

The tensions around this issue were shown in early 2021 when residents vandalized and destroyed preparatory structures that the municipality had put in place with the intention of constructing a playground and education centre. One resident looking on remarked that 'Israel kills children and now wants to build playgrounds for them'.[59] Zughayer told me that the 'municipality demolished buildings to build parks without consulting with us because they want to build settlements'. He suggested this is why Palestinians vandalize and destroy them. He adds that this is part of a larger plan to build a tunnel under Qalandiya military checkpoint and expropriate land from areas in Jerusalem, including Kufr ʿAqab.[60] This appears to be accurate – in November 2021, the local municipal planning committee in Jerusalem approved the building of 9,000 units for Ultra-Orthodox Jews in Qalandia area, which lies adjacent to Kufr ʿAqab.[61] Many Palestinian families will be evicted if the plan is implemented, and Israel postponed the plan after the European Union and the United States objected.

Israel confiscated land from the village to build settlements and a military base, and demolished Palestinian homes to build roads and connect settlements (ARIJ, 2012: 17).[62] One interviewee observes Israel has opened centres at the checkpoint that will deal with Interior Ministry and national insurance issues – in their view, this is a prelude to the area being separated from Jerusalem.[63] This is also the view of Ola Awad-Shakhshir, the minister of Palestinian Central Bureau of Statistics, who is from Kufr ʿAqab.[64]

This is also consistent with the 'Greater Jerusalem' bill that MK Yoav Kisch and Minister Yisrael Katz (both Likud) proposed to the Knesset in 2017 and Netanyahu's wider annexation plan and the long-established desire to attain 'a maximum of land with a minimum of Arabs' (Benvenisti, 1995: 53).[65] Under the terms of this proposal, Jerusalem's boundaries will be expanded so that illegal settlements (and more than 200, 000 settlers) fall within Israel's sovereignty.

Residents endure poor infrastructure and a lack of services. Zughayer notes a lack of urban planning and safety regulations, and claims this is a serious problem that could escalate into an even worse one in the future. He adds that residents, some of whom live in fourteen-storey building with water tanks and solar panels on the roofs, will be particularly vulnerable in the event of an earthquake.[66] Their fate is subject to the will of others (the situation of those 'who must live and those who must die', in the words of Foucault, 2003: 239)[67] and they are condemned to live an 'animal life' (Mbembe, 2003: 24).[68]

In Kufr ʿAqab, there is lawlessness and a security vacuum. The Israeli police only intervenes to collect taxes or fines. Disputes and breaches of the law are arbitrated and resolved at the family level although on rare occasions, as on Saturday 2 January 2021, when three family members were shot dead during a family feud, the PA is invited to intervene. However, this can only occur under coordination, as Palestinians in Kufr 'Aqab have Jerusalem IDs.[69] But in other respects, it is preferable to Jerusalem. Jamal Juma, for example, observes that while it is 'suffocating', it is 'less stressful' because here it is possible to avoid house demolitions, arbitrary checks by soldiers or police, 'incredibly expensive' taxes and home raids at night.[70] Other interviewees cited the expensive real estate in Jerusalem, along with the costs of owning or renting. One claims the Arnona (municipal tax) in Jerusalem city for a smaller size apartment is more than triple the amount required for a larger one in Kufr 'Aqab. Palestinians also require permission to build a house or an apartment and this is subject to a long and expensive ten-step process that requires municipal coordination and approval.[71]

All interviewees complained of a lack of urban planning and buildings that lacked safety measures, regulations or proper electricity, sewage and water services. They tended to focus on these factors, in addition to lawlessness, even after I explained that my research was focused on coronavirus in Kufr 'Aqab. All interviewees complained about things like garbage collection, unpaved roads, a lack of sanitation/sewage system and poor wastewater drainage. Outsourcing of garbage collection to private companies[72] and the expensive and time-consuming use of legal recourse to address problems with water and sewage were other concerns.[73]

Although Israel's service provision for Palestinians in the Jerusalem muncipality is inadequate, it resists PA interference. B'Tselem explains:

> In July 2015, Ir Amim petitioned the Jerusalem muncipality on the residents' behalf demanding that roads in these neighborhoods be repaired. The petition described grave neglect, including an almost complete lack of services. The roads are in disrepair, sewage and electricity infrastructure is deficient and there is a shortage of schools, sidewalks and playgrounds. There is also a lack of vital facilities such as mother and child clinics and mail distribution and fire-fighting services. The municipality does not provide cleaning services, which are instead supplied by the PA (2017).[74]

During the winter, a lack of rain water drainage also creates many ponds. Interviewees complained contractors of unregulated buildings did not provide proper infrastructure, leading people to steal electricity and water.[75] An additional complication is that some buildings are built on land that belongs to diaspora Palestinians.[76] Dajani, De Leo and AlKhalidi (2013) suggest that informal urbanization and the lack of regulations are intended by Israel because this will ultimately enable it to wash its hands of the neighbourhood.[77]

Zughayar suggests that it is a priority to first solve the sewage, water and garbage problems by putting in place basic services, like clean water and proper sewage drainage. He indicated he would seek recourse through Israeli courts. However, he maintains that even though the movement of sewage would spread disease across the wall, Israel would still be reluctant to address the issue because it is a racist state.[78]

The problem is further compounded by Israel's control of water resources, and more specifically the restrictions it imposes on the drilling of wells and its banning of the installation of water structures (Al-Tamimi, 2021).[79] Mekorot, the Israeli water supply company that controls the distribution of water to the PA,[80] also provides a limited supply that results in shortages and can be cut off for days (Israeli settlements nearby experience no shortages and indeed enjoy an unlimited supply of water),[81] and this forces residents to buy extra water tanks and trucked water at very high prices. In contrast to the Beit Hanina area, which is not cut off from Jerusalem by a checkpoint or wall, Kufr 'Aqab receives its water supply from the PA, which purchases water at an expensive rate.[82] After the Second *Intifada*, officials from the Palestinian water authority are not allowed to enter and so, whenever there is an issue or problem, Israel hires a contractor from Jerusalem instead, with international donors meeting the costs of maintenance and/or installation.[83] This fundamental inequality is enshrined in the Oslo Accords, which only allow Palestinians to access less than one-fifth (17 per cent) of the aquifer water. Selby observes:

Overall, it was Israel which was the chief beneficiary of the Oslo II water accords: without sacrificing control over water resources or having to forego its discriminatory water policy, it nonetheless managed to transfer a range of administrative and financial burdens to the Palestinians and their international donors - chiefly the responsibility for rehabilitating water networks and improving water supplies, and the responsibility for ensuring Palestinian payment for water supplies. (2005: 5)[84]

The impermanence of Kufr 'Aqab's population, which is constantly changing and shifting, is another defining feature. Ir Amin observes:

[The separation wall] created two waves of migration. The first consisted primarily of middle-class residents who lived in the suburbs outside the municipal boundaries of the city, where they had moved to avoid the neglect and severe building restrictions inside East Jerusalem. Many of these residents, estimated to number tens of thousands, fearing the negative impact of the Barrier on their way of life and their residency status, subsequently moved back into the core neighborhoods of East Jerusalem, accepting far worse living conditions than they had been able to enjoy in the suburbs. This wave created intense pressure on the already limited housing market in East Jerusalem, precipitating a second wave of migration by poorer residents who left neighborhoods within the city and moved to Jerusalem neighborhoods beyond the Barrier where they could secure relatively cheap and available housing. (2015: 25)[85]

Some residents are effectively trapped here. One interviewee is unable to leave because her husband does not have a Jerusalem ID, and she is afraid to after two of her sisters had their residency revoked when they moved to other countries. Although she pays taxes and national insurance, they have no rights and receive no services in return. There are no parks or playgrounds for her children. Although she would prefer to enrol her children in a school in the city of Jerusalem, she cannot do this because crossing the checkpoint is dangerous, and there is a danger they will be exposed to violence. The schools in Kufr 'Aqab are low quality.[86] Another interviewee confirmed this but chose to send his children to school in Jerusalem city, despite them seeing shootings and arrests at checkpoints. He told me, 'it is about choosing something at the expense of another'.[87]

Those with Jerusalem IDs remain here to prevent them from being revoked – one interviewee told me that she refused a citizenship in another country, with more benefits, in order to retain her ID. This is just one illustration of how Palestinians will endure a host of predicaments and obstacles in order to prove the city is their 'centre of life' and remain there. One Kufr 'Aqab resident, who is waiting for his application for Jerusalem residency to be confirmed, explains:

> Israeli National Insurance representatives pay us visits to check if our 'center of life' is within Jerusalem municipality as part of my application process to Jerusalem ID. These visits were interrupted due to corona virus, but resumed recently. Few weeks ago, I was at my son's house in Ramallah and representative showed up and accused me of not living in Jerusalem. I told him that was only vising and he accompanied me to my house in Kufr 'Aqab to check. He started to compare electricity consumption and food amount in the refrigerators in the home of Kufr 'Aqab and the one in Ramallah. He concluded that my center of life seemed to be more in Ramallah. I tried to explain, but he just said, 'we will see'.[88]

His friend, who lived outside the Jerusalem area as this meant he did not need to travel for work, was also subject to a 'centre of life' investigation. He used various methods of disguise, including putting a different name on his house, parking his car on a different street and taking care when entering and leaving his home. However, he was caught after an Israeli national insurance representative followed him and took photos of him to prove that his 'centre of life' was actually Ramallah. His friend had to move back to Jerusalem. Another resident told me that 'national insurance representatives also collect information from neighbours, supermarkets and shops'[89] Israel also seeks to 'tame' resisting activists and those who fail to prove the city is their 'centre of life' by withholding their national and health insurance entitlements.

One resident spoke of how 'we live here just to wait' (quoted in Ashley, 2018)[90] and another referred to a 'no man's land' where the municipality had stopped providing (already basic) services after the Second *Intifada*.[91] A sense of uncertainty[92] and an absence of purpose are pervasive here. Abu Hatoum speaks of how the residents exist in 'a deep suspension of no-state' where they are '[k]ept at the frontier of settler-colonialism' and are 'suspended in time' (2021: 104).[93]

One interviewee explained to me how Palestinians with Jerusalem ID have to be careful and alert all the time because 'every information might affect your eligibility for Jerusalem ID'.[94] Hamayel, Hammoudeh and Welchman (2017) present the 'centre of life' policy, checkpoints and the wall as biopolitical tools that are inflicted on Palestinians in Kufr 'Aqab.[95] Each of these measures, in addition to the granting of permits,[96] is part of a system of surveillance that seeks to discipline and control (Weizman, 2007; Halper, 2015).[97] The residents inhabit Foucault's panoptican prison,[98] where they are not just subject to external influence but also internalize surveillance and self-discipline.

Health is part of this biopolitical spectrum of surveillance. Spouses of Jerusalem ID holders are entitled to register for Israeli health insurance when they initiate the unification procedure and can, subject to payment, obtain a permit after proving the city is their 'centre of life'. In 2016, Israel made it mandatory for Palestinians with a green West Bank ID who were married to a Jerusalemites to obtain health insurance. Khalid told me: 'I never received a letter regarding the new law that required health insurance for my wife. I only learnt about it through Facebook later. I had to pay 7, 850 USD to insure my wife and a monthly payment of 90 USD'.[99] Israeli health insurance companies also began to ask for a back charge payment, despite the spouses never receiving any medical services. A 2016 appeal by the Society of St Yves to the Supreme Court did result in the payment being reduced, although this only came into force in 2021,[100] and residents complain that the companies continue to ignore it. This policy is part of Israel's discriminatory measures that seek to dispossess Palestinians and force them into enclaves.[101] Families forced to reside here because of mixed

IDs are subject to different biopolitical tools that control them and exclude them from Jerusalem (Hamayel, Hammoudeh and Welchman, 2017).[102] They must also live with the continual fear that their residency will be revoked on 'good conduct' grounds. And in 2021, Israel, in the wider context of unrest around the Al-Aqsa mosque, revoked the health insurance of sixteen former Palestinian prisoners and their families on the grounds they did not reside in Jerusalem and the city was not their 'centre of life'.[103]

If only one spouse has a Jerusalem ID, mothers are required to deliver their child in a hospital in the city for them to obtain residency. Women must therefore cross the checkpoint, where they experience violence in many cases. Women with a West Bank ID must first obtain a permit to enter Jerusalem. One study observes:

> [O]ne woman asked her doctor to induce her birth in line with the duration of a permit allowance given to her husband so she could ensure he would be able to witness the birth of their child. Having understood the difficulty in obtaining a permit for her husband in time for childbirth, the doctor empathized with the couple and agreed to an induced labor. (Hammoudeh, Hamayel and Welchman, 2016: 43)[104]

Unsurprisingly, given their experiences, residents now warn their children not to endure the same hardships in the hope this will produce the required permit. One interviewee told me that 'Jerusalemites now advice their children not to get married to a West Bank ID holder to avoid such painful experience and difficulties'.[105]

Responding to the pandemic in Kufr 'Aqab

During the pandemic, there was pervasive chaos and lawlessness in Kufr 'Aqab. Palestinians from 'locked down' areas came for weddings, parties and shopping. One interviewee notes: 'Kufr 'Aqab never closed down and remained open all the time. The only time shops in Kufr

'Aqab closed, was for the general strike of May 18th, in response to Palestinians in Israel call[106] and it was a voluntary action.'[107]

One interviewee notes:

> During feast and holiday seasons the neighbourhood remains open until 5.00 in the morning. Many traders from Ramallah open businesses in Kufr Aqab to avoid paying taxes. No one is concerned with corona, all shops are opened, it is crowded and there are no preventive measure. My family and I are cautious and take protective measures, but it is difficult among the chaos. My son became infected with corona, although we are careful.[108]

Interviewees observed that compliance with pandemic 'best practice' is non-existent in Kufr 'Aqab and were only aware of a few ineffective PA initiatives. One noted tests were not available and that it was easier to get tested in Ramallah.[109] Residents without national insurances, spouse of Jerusalem ID holders without health and social security rights, outsourced medical services and unqualified doctors were among the health-related challenges that confronted the community in Kufr 'Aqab.[110]

Meanwhile, Israel refused to vaccinate Palestinians, which is consistent with its more general refusal to meet its responsibilities as an occupying power. After 8,000 Palestinian health workers tested positive, the WHO asked Israel to vaccinate Palestinian health workers and keep the Palestinian heath system afloat.[111] Israel refused and claimed it did not have enough vaccines for Israelis.[112] Yuli Edelstein, Israel's health minister, denied his country had any legal obligation to vaccinate Palestinians. He said:

> As far as vaccination is concerned I think it is Israel's obligation first and foremost to its citizens – they pay taxes for that, don't they? If it is the responsibility of the Israeli health ministry to take care of the Palestinians, what exactly is the responsibility of the Palestinian health minister – to take care of the dolphins in the Mediterranean?[113]

When the virus broke out, Israel did not include Palestinian Jerusalemites in its response plan. Kufr 'Aqab and Palestinians in the Jerusalem municipality did not receive any additional services. This was a particular issue as the majority of residents of Kufr 'Aqab who hold Jerusalem IDs have to travel through the Qalandia checkpoint to reach Ramallah which could, taking congestion into account, consume up to two hours. During the pandemic, the residents were left without direct access to health services in Jerusalem. When Israel imposed a lockdown after the virus broke out, residents of Kufr 'Aqab were, without exception or notice, prevented from crossing the checkpoint and entering Jerusalem.[114]

Israel also blamed Palestinians for spreading the virus. Professor Ronni Gamzu, who was appointed in July 2020 as National Coronavirus Project Coordinator and Director of the Special Operations Control Center likened the spread of the virus among Palestinian citizens of Israel to 'a mass terror attack' and accused them of an assortment of sins ('gatherings, riots, parties, complacency, apathy') and of harbouring a false belief that the virus would not hurt them.[115]

This reflected the 'securitization' of the pandemic. In responding to Palestinian protests at Al-Aqsa Mosque in May 2021, Israel used the pretext of tracking the spread of Covid-19 to target activists. For example, Israeli intelligence staff sent threatening text messages to Palestinians during protests in Jerusalem. One read: 'You have been identified to have taken part in violent acts at Al-Aqsa Mosque. We will hold you accountable.'[116] This is deliberately ambiguous, as it is far from clear what 'hold you accountable' does, or even could, entail. Shalhoub-Kevorkian observes:

> This politics of fear and surveillance leaves the colonized constantly insecure, particularly because they are unable to interpret or appropriately handle the many complex symbols, forms of rhetoric and visualities of the colonialist. They are constantly on guard, not knowing when and how they have crossed the line, and of course they are always guilty. (2015: 23)[117]

And he adds this 'politics of fear' '[can] simultaneously [be used to] include and exclude, eliminate and incorporate, assimilate and reject, while producing new categories and modes of sameness and otherness that serve to naturalize settler dominance' (2015: 7).[118]

Israel also deliberately obstructed the Palestinian response. When the PA tried to test Jerusalemites, Israel refused and closed the testing center.[119] It was subsequently impossible to confirm the extent to which the virus had spread. Zughayer cooperated with Adalah, the Legal Center for Arab Minority Rights, to petition the Israeli Supreme Court on its failure to provide testing and other services to 150,000 Palestinians within the municipality and beyond the wall, including to residents of Kufr 'Aqab and the Shuafat refugee camp.[120],[121] The Court responded by ordering Israel to open testing centres 'beyond the wall'.[122] However, Adalah (which requested this measure) claimed it was necessary but not sufficient and had called for additional measures that would help to identify the extent of virus spread 'beyond the wall'.[123]

In early 2021, Adalah responded to the lack of vaccination centres in Kufr 'Aqab by forwarding a letter to the Israeli Health Ministry and Israeli health organizations and, in referring to their responsibility for administering vaccines, asked them to provide vaccinations to residents 'beyond the wall'.[124] Israel then opened vaccination centres near the wall. However, Jamal Juma claims this was only to benefit Palestinians 'beyond the wall' who work in Israel.

Uptake remained limited because it is easier for Kufr 'Aqab residents to be tested in Ramallah[125] and because many Palestinians avoid testing because of suspicions about the trace system and the isolation requirements. Interviewees attributed vaccine hesitancy to a fear that they would be used for medical experiments, in the same way that Palestinian prisoners were rumoured to be.[126] There were rumours about sterilization[127] and the use of expired vaccines, and this is why residents 'beyond the wall preferred to be vaccinated in centers that serve both Jews and Arabs'. This hesitancy was, however, eventually overcome – Zughayer claimed this was because vaccination was a prerequisite for prisoner visits,[128] while another interviewee asserted it was an administrative requirement of the Israeli Ministry of Interior. She insisted, however, on receiving the vaccination in Jerusalem city, because she believed the one at the checkpoint was expired.[129],[130]

Israel's (in)actions clearly recall the UN's warning that the pandemic is an additional threat to indigenous communities that have the potential to gravely impact their livelihoods and economy. There is a clear overlap between the experiences of these indigenous communities and Palestinians in the pandemic, and this is why it is crucial for Palestinians to acknowledge the UN's recommendation that the representatives, leaders and traditional authorities of indigenous peoples be included 'in the planning and design of health services and responses to the COVID-19 pandemic as well as in dealing with its repercussions'.[131]

The PA's role in Kufr 'Aqab should also be considered. One resident told me that widespread disregard for pandemic 'best practice' reflected the fact that people do not respect the PA.[132] Jamal Juma notes this may be due to politicization and observes that Fatah, with the support of the PA, sought to use these initiatives for its own political purposes, and also frustrated efforts by other political parties to provide support to communities.[133] He also suggests indifference to the pandemic had a class dimension and noted that people lived in a dire situation where the virus was the least of their worries. He referred to chaos and continual shooting, and suggested the virus was a priority for the middle and upper classes who had time to worry about their lives whereas the lower classes are more concerned with meeting daily needs.[134]

Although the PA cannot enforce isolation, it coordinates with Israel and provides information about numbers and data on positive cases. However, as one interviewee notes, the reluctance to self-report will distort the data.[135] There are clearly a number of incentives in this regard – if a Palestinian tests positive, then Israel will cancel the whole family's permits; one interviewee said he was not allowed to cross the checkpoint to get his second dose of the vaccine after his son was registered as positive;[136] and there is also no furlough scheme. Accordingly, whenever family members of workers in Israel show Covid-19 symptoms, they will avoid testing.

One resident spoke of no data on Kufr 'Aqab and of being unable to identify how Israel or the PA defined Jerusalem. They also complained that PA's reports are broad and only sometimes include details.[137] Although the Palestinian Ministry of Health publishes the total cases of coronavirus cases registered in Palestinian areas (including Jerusalem), it is not clear which parts of Jerusalem are included. Dr Salwa Najjab told me that data on Jerusalem is often missing from the reports and is only available when Israel provides it.

Adalah observes:

> The lack of published data concerning Arab towns and villages in Israel is not only an example of structural discrimination against the Palestinian Arab minority in Israel, but also a major public health hazard for the population in Israel and the OPT as a whole. Additionally, from March to early May 2020, the daily MOH update excluded data on dozens of towns with a population of under 5,000 residents;24 the data on these towns were presented together, with no division according to town or nationality. (2020: 10)[138]

This lack of usable information has a clear parallel in the treatment (or non-treatment) of native American communities in census collection. Abigail Echo-Hawk, director of the urban Indian health institute and the chief research officer for the Seattle Indian Health Board, observes: 'I see being eliminated in the data as an ongoing part of the continuing genocide of American Indians and Alaska Natives. If you eliminate us in the data, we no longer exist.'[139]

Dr Ola Awad-Shakhshir, minister of PCBS (Palestinian Central Bureau of Statistics), told me[140] that 'Israel doesn't allow Palestinians to conduct population census in Jerusalem. During the first census conducted in 1997, workers were arrested. Following Oslo and in 1997 Knesset passed a legislation that bans Palestinians from conducting [a] census in East Jerusalem' (see NYT, 1997).[141]

The PCBS observes:

> The law [1997 Knesset legislation that prohibits Palestinian from conducting a census in East Jerusalem] was passed within 24 hours only, without passing the three-reading procedure as laws usually enacted in the occupying state do. The Palestinians demonstrated

resolve and did not give way to these measures and they continued to work secretly in full swing in Jerusalem through various possible means (Palestinian Central Bureau of Statistics, 2020: 8).[142]

In 2017, Israel accused seventeen Palestinians of collecting data for the census and arrested them.[143] Awad-Shakhshir explained how the PCBS divides Jerusalem into two areas (J1 and J2), when collecting data for technical reasons. She told me:

> Israel defines the borders of Jerusalem and there are areas within the wall and areas beyond it. The areas beyond the wall and within municipal boundaries of the city, such as Kufr Aqab and the Shuafat refugee camp became like other areas outside the city's borders, such as A-Ram, Al-Izzariyya, Abu Dis and Area C. When we collect data on the impact of COVID 19, we are obliged, for statistical purposes, to recognize these areas have a different economy and services. (also see PCBS, 2021: 36)[144]

Mallard et al. observe that the lack of data on how Covid-19 affects indigenous people hinders related decision-making and also reduces the likelihood that appropriately tailored approaches will emerge (2021: 4).[145] This should be factored into the UN's warning that service inadequacies could result in high case rates in indigenous communities[146] and should also be considered in combination with Alfred's (2005) observation that colonial dispossession produces poorer native health outcomes and disease rates that exceed those recorded in the settler community.[147]

In the absence of an effective and coordinated response from either Israel or the PA, Zughayer observes that local neighbourhood committees organized campaigns with the aim of providing popular education on Covid-19 and necessary safety measures.[148] However, when compared against the pre-Oslo period, such initiatives were minimal in scope.[149] Colonization and neoliberalism have created a detached leadership and weakened political parties, with the consequence that both have a weak ability to lead popular mobilization and establish a basis for solidarity in the face of the challenges that confront Kufr 'Aqab.

Conclusion

Israel's actions and activities in Kufr 'Aqab are an outgrowth of broader policies in East Jerusalem that seek to manipulate demographic realities and establish a Jewish advantage in what Israel considers to be its eternal and indivisible capital. The construction of Israel's 'separation' wall has instituted an arrangement in which a surplus population has been consigned to the outer reaches of Jerusalem and forced to endure a kind of administrative purgatory in which they are subject to assorted indignities, arbitrary restrictions and impositions.

And yet some residents have chosen to live here, viewing it as necessary in order to acquire required bureaucratic permissions and to find respite from Israel's repeated harassment in East Jerusalem. However, their existence here is a grim one, characterized by near non-existent services, administrative inertia and arbitrary restrictions and intrusions. This is a 'bare life', in which there is not even the partial compensation of social solidarity and support – neighbours are strangers, and to be regarded with the same reserve and suspicion as the colonial occupier. This attested to the 'securitization' of the pandemic.

In every sense, including the economic, political and social, Kufr 'Aqab's population are pushed to the margins and excluded. However, this does not imply that the colonizer is entirely disinterested in them, as its extensive and intrusive apparatus of surveillance and oversight attests. Indeed, the 'centre of life' policy clearly establishes that Israel is intimately interested in every movement and action of residents, and is predisposed to interrogate them in minute and exacting detail. Residents are required to justify their existence and prove to the satisfaction of the colonial authority that they should be permitted to remain. Here, the Israeli 'gaze' extends far and wide, simultaneously acknowledging, registering and permitting.

Residents are not, however, regarded as objects of concerns but rather as objects of potential threat or danger. On the basis of extensive past experience, they know better than to expect anything from a colonizer that 'gives nothing away', and indeed, they would perhaps expect Israel to destroy testing centres or fail to take active measures to enable Palestinians to access healthcare. However, unlike elsewhere in the West Bank, it appears that Israel was willing to take limited measures to ensure that Palestinians who worked in Israel were vaccinated. In this context, the persistence of rumours and mistrust was clearly to be expected.

They are fully aware that the colonizer's interest in them extends only as far as their potential to hinder or subvert colonial designs. Through their (non) existence in a sealed-off administrative purgatory, they have similarly come to understand that the PA is not in a position to meet their needs and requirements, whether as a result of a lack of will, resources and/or legal entitlement. Israel, for its part, jealously guards its entitlements here and, in accordance with established precedent, only permits the PA to act when it sees an opportunity to 'outsource' unwanted tasks. Residents, who endure a chaotic, uncertain and precarious existence, in any case long ago learned to rely on themselves. There is no law here and no security, and only a 'bare life' to aspire to.

In common with the Gaza Strip, poor sewage and wastewater disposal, in addition to limited access to water, crowded living conditions and medical services, left Kufr 'Aqab residents exposed to the pandemic. However, interviewees tended to speak of them as challenges in their own right rather than as factors that could directly contribute to virus spread, which spoke volumes about their order of priorities. If anything, social life gained a new dimension in the pandemic, as Palestinians travelled to Kufr 'Aqab from other parts of the West Bank. Otherwise, the lives of residents continued as normal.

Life here is defined by a lack of purpose and so it would clearly be counter-intuitive to expect residents to collectively mobilize in response to the challenges they face. Instead, in accordance with the concept of 'no state', it would seem more likely that action/s would be without purpose or initiative. Here the difficulties of political mobilization noted elsewhere in the West Bank are intensified and multiplied to a higher degree. They intersect with class and politicization, which also appear as 'limiting factors' of political agency and activism.

While the PA had a limited ability to alter this or produce political mobilization, it could conceivably have helped to produce a more effective public response by assuming a more proactive role in collecting and distributing data. In this regard, both gaps in the data and shortcomings in public messaging (which contributed to ignorance and scepticism) were identified as important factors by interviewees. In doing so, it would encounter the main factors that currently impede its work, which include the fragmentation of Palestinian land, the emergence and consolidation of Bantustans (see Yiftachel, 2009; Benvenisti, 2010) and a sub-divided Palestinian population (Hilal, 2015).[150]

In this regard, both gaps in the data and shortcomings in public messaging (which contributed to ignorance and scepticism) were identified as important factors by interviewees. However, as elsewhere in the West Bank, it was poorly suited to perform this role, not least because its commitment to security cooperation has left it dangerously detached from domestic constituencies. This adds a new dimension to the critique of the PA's role in the pandemic response.

Life and death on the margins

The pandemic in Jalazone refugee camp

Introduction

In 27 June 2018, Prince William, the duke of Cambridge, visited Jalazone Camp as part of his Middle East tour and told his audience of refugees that 'you have not been forgotten'. As he was leaving, one Palestinian reminded him of the Balfour Declaration's promise to establish a Jewish national home in Palestine.[1] This is just one example of how the Palestinian past remains intertwined in the present. Tanous further affirms that this 'example of deception and trickery' produced 'an ugly battle that started sixty years ago and we do not see an end to it in the near future' (1982: 57).[2]

UNRWA, the United Nations Relief and Works Agency for Palestine Refugees in the Near East, defines Palestinian refugees as 'people whose normal place of residence was Palestine between June 1946 and May 1948, who lost their homes and livelihoods to the 1948 Arab-Israeli conflict'.[3] It estimates there are currently 5.6 million Palestinian refugees (see Figure 5.1), who can trace their current situation back to the *Nakba* of 1948, when around 750,000 Palestinians, or 80 per cent of the total population of historical Palestine, were forced to relocate to the West Bank, Gaza Strip and neighbouring and international countries.

UNRWA was formed in December 1949 to advocate on behalf of, assist and protect Palestinian refugees. This was made harder by the fact that the categorization of these refugees and the estimation of their numbers has always been highly politicized, as Zureik notes:

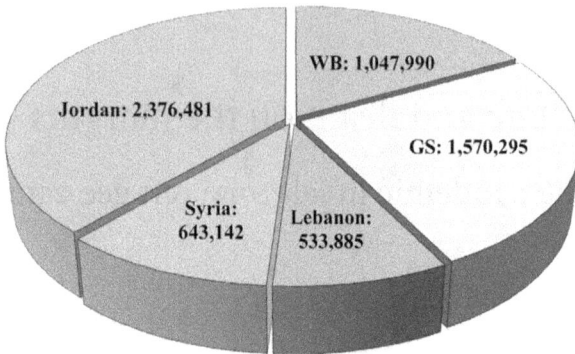

Figure 5.1 UNRWA-Total RPs by Area (1/2/2019). *Source*: The Palestine Strategic Report, 2021: 93. (Saleh, Mohsen Mohammad (ed.) (2021). The Palestine Strategic Report 2018–2019. Al-Zaytouna Centre for Studies & Consultations Beirut-Lebanon.)

> Refugees who ended up in places other than UNRWA's so-called five areas of operations (Syria, Lebanon, Jordan, the West Bank, and Gaza) did not appear in UNRWA's registry. Similarly, those who were internally displaced (present- absentee) in Palestine during the fighting in 1948 and 1949, and remain displaced to this day in what became Israel, do not appear in UNRWA's refugee count, even though UNRWA did include them initially until Israel terminated the Agency's jurisdiction over them in 1952. (2001: 219)[4]

More recently, the future of the agency has been called into question by funding reductions that could gravely impact the refugees and their living conditions by robbing them of their only legal international witness.[5] The Trump administration tried to pressurize the PA by cutting its funding for the agency in 2018, despite being fully aware this would negatively impact the agency's education and health services (Cook, 2018).[6] This was part of a more general departure from international law, as the Trump administration's positions on the Palestinian Right of Return (Beaumont and Holmes, 2018)[7] and the Syrian Golan Heights (recognized as part of Israel in April 2019) demonstrated.

However, even though the Biden administration reversed this decision in April 2021[8] and provided the PA with $15 million to combat

Covid-19, its future remains uncertain.[9] Precisely one year later, its commissioner-general, who has suggested it is 'close to collapse',[10] was forced to suggest partnerships as a way of protecting essential services and rights.[11]

The Palestinian refugee 'problem' is widely acknowledged to be a root cause of the Israeli–Palestinian conflict and the right of return is established in international law. However, after the Palestinian leadership accepted the Oslo agreements, their status became subject to negotiations, and this appeared to indicate the Palestinian leadership was willing to compromise on this matter: far from being acknowledged as central to the conflict, the refugees now appeared to be regarded as one among a number of (equally important) 'final status' issues.[12] Whereas the Palestinian 'problem' had previously been synonymous with the Palestinian refugees driven from their homes in 1948, the political emphasis now shifted to the Palestinians (of the West Bank and Gaza Strip) who had lived under occupation since 1967.

In part, this was an acknowledgement of political realities, as Israeli governments have repeatedly refused to acknowledge the Right of Return in any meaningful way. For example, they never recognized UNSCR 194, which

> Resolves that refugees wishing to return to their homes and live at peace with their neighbors should be permitted to do so at the earliest practicable date, and that compensation should be paid for the property of those choosing not to return and for loss of or damage to property, which, under principles of international law or inequity, should be made good by the Governments or authorities responsible.[13] P. 8

In 1951 Moshe Sharett,[14] Israel's then foreign minister, said:

> An account already exists between us and the Arab world: the account of the compensation that accrues to the Arabs who left the territory of Israel and abandoned their property … . The act that has now been perpetrated by the Kingdom of Iraq … forces us to link the two accounts … . We will take into account the value of the Jewish property that has been frozen in Iraq when calculating the compensation that

we have undertaken to pay the Arabs who abandoned property in Israel. (quoted in Shenhav, 1999: 605)[15]

Khalidi observes that the text of the 1978 Camp David Accords suggested the 'refugee problem'[16] could be appropriately dealt with by Israel and Egypt and 'other interested parties'. As in the Balfour Declaration, '[t]here was no mention of the Palestinians themselves' (2013: 6).[17] Furthermore, on 22 January1978, Carter formally informed Menachem Begin, the Israeli prime minister, that his references to 'Palestinians' or 'Palestinian people' alluded to Palestinian Arabs (2013: 6). In more recent times, the United States has reassured Israel that it will only enter into peace negotiations with its approval (2013: 8).

In the 2000 Camp David negotiations, the Israeli government put forward a 'satisfactory solution' which would allow a few thousand refugees to return and attempted to use this 'concession' to obtain compensation for Jewish refugees who had been expelled from Arab countries.

Sayigh reflects:

> Meanwhile, nothing has been offered to the refugees who fled or were expelled in 1948, to the hundreds of thousands of new refugees from the war in 1967, or to the victims of the 'silent expulsions' that have followed until the present. The only step towards a resolution of their miserable plight was at the Taba negotiations, which partially recognized UN Resolution 194, calling for return or compensation. The tentative agreement at Taba would have allowed return of Palestinians to the new state of Palestine, and some symbolic return to Israel that would not affect the 'demographic balance', a permanent concern in a state based on ethnic predominance. But for now, even those avenues are closed. (2008: 193)[18]

In Israel, the Right of Return 'touches on deep-seated fears [...] regarding the legitimacy and permanence of the entire Zionist enterprise, as well as the Arab-Jewish demographic balance within Palestine' (Khalidi, 1992: 29).[19] Masalha notes this concern with Palestinian demography and land was established from an early stage, and was 'at the heart of the Zionist transfer mind-set and secret transfer plans of the 1930s and 1940s' (2002: 77).[20]

And we should link this blindness to Palestinian rights to Jewish supremacy. In 2018, the Knesset passed the Jewish Nation-State Basic Law, which establishes: 'The State of Israel is the national state of the Jewish people, in which it exercises its natural, cultural, and historic right to self-determination [and adds] [e]xercising the right to national self-determination in the State of Israel is unique to the Jewish people' (Adalah, 2020).[21] In referring to this law in a 2019 cabinet meeting, Netanyahu further clarified that Israel 'is the nation-state, not of all its citizens, but only of the Jewish people'.[22]

This chapter provides a case study of the situation of Palestinian refugees in Jalazone and provides an insight into the situation of Palestinian refugees in the oPt. In doing so, it addresses UNRWA's concept of a common suffering among Palestinian refugees while acknowledging the specificity of each refugee camp.

Before the pandemic, Palestine refugees were already among the most vulnerable communities in the Middle East. Measures taken to mitigate and suppress the spread of the virus have exacerbated this situation, and have severely impacted lives and livelihoods (UNRWA, 2020: 5).[23]

Palestinian refugees suffer from poor living conditions that are aggravated by the virus. As the case study will demonstrate, it is not just difficult, but impossible, for refugees to take required safety measures. Given this, it is hardly surprising that Covid-19 deaths in Palestinian refugee camps in Lebanon are three times the national level.[24] In February 2021, 200 of 5,000 infected refugees in Lebanese camps died of the virus.[25] A recent study has also shown how efforts to combat the virus in Lebanon's refugee camps have been constrained by poor conditions, poverty (both work and property-related), lawlessness and mental health issues.[26] A number of these challenges confront Palestinian refugees more generally.

Jalazone refugee camp

The camp was established in 1949 to accommodate those who had been forced to leave what later became Israel. The camp is mainly located in

Area B, although parts, including UNRWA's boys' and girls' schools are
near an Israeli settlement and therefore fall within Area C.[27] The UN
agency observes:

> UNRWA schools and students are frequently exposed to tear gas,
> sound bombs and other forms of weaponry, including already on two
> occasions this year. Such incidents can lead to fatalities and injuries
> as they have in the past. They are very stressful and disruptive to the
> education and development of the children and can have long-term
> impacts on the[ir] physical and mental well-being.[28]

The nearby Beit El settlement, which was built in 1977, infringes
and intrudes on daily life in the camp. Israel constructed a wall that
separated the settlement from the main road, cutting one Palestinian
family off from the rest of the camp. Settlers also frequently block
the road, which forces camp residents to take a longer road to access
Ramallah, the nearest city, for work or to access different services.

'Multiple powers' turn the camp's residents into the 'living dead'
(2003: 40).[29] They are 'in pain' all the time (Mbembe, 2003: 39)[30] and
are continually pushed towards becoming 'bare life' (Agamben, 1998:
81–6).[31] One camp resident observes '[t]he Israeli army invades the
Camp daily and soldiers vandalize homes and arrest people . . . all this
affects the economy'[32]. And another adds that the settlement causes
almost daily friction with the Israeli army.[33] Even during the pandemic,
the Israeli army did not stop its intrusions – Dalashi observes: 'Arrests
never stopped and during the peak of the virus, soldiers wore gloves
and masks to enter homes. They dressed persons under arrest in white
suits, and then threw them in isolated prisons for 14 days.'[34] B'Tselem
observes that it 'is difficult to quantify the overall impact of the travel
restriction because camp residents state they prefer not to leave the
camp unless absolutely necessary, as they can never know when the
road will suddenly be closed'.[35]

It is not merely the direct impacts, but also the perpetual uncertainty,
that imposes itself on the camp's residents. Quite clearly, this is no life at
all, and indeed more closely resembles a living death. Residents inhabit

'death-worlds' and are the 'living dead' (Mbembe, 2003: 40).[36] They endure a 'bare life' in a 'state of exception' where 'everything is possible' (Agamben, 1998: 172),[37] bringing to mind Agamben's observation that those who have been banned are 'not, in fact, simply set outside the law and made indifferent to it, but rather *abandoned* [emphasis in original] by it, that is, exposed and threatened on the threshold in which life and law, outside and inside, become indistinguishable' (1998: 28).[38]

And this brings to mind Shalhoub-Kevorkian's 'industry of fear [that] aims at sociocide, which attacks the social fabric and daily life of the colonized, their land, their property and their politics of truth. She clarifies that under its conditions, "*the colonized are forever questioning what is happening around them*'" [emphasis added] (2015: 10–11).[39] This reiterates that (in)security is not an objective condition but is rather something that the coloniser imposes on the Native (Fanon, 1963: 53–4).[40] In continually invoking 'security' as some kind of sanctified right, Israel consciously and deliberately inflicting various forms of insecurity on Palestinians. Through 'multiple powers' (Foucault, 1995: 198–9),[41] it therefore commits itself to a 'spacio-cidal' project (Hanafi, 2009)[42] that fragments land and restricts movement

UNRWA, the PA and Western donors

Jalazone residents view their situation as temporary and assert their right to return to their homes. They therefore concur with powerful actors in the international system who, as Agamben observes, view refugee status as 'a temporary condition that should lead either to naturalization or to repatriation'. However, there is a clear difference in the expectation of refugees that the belated recognition of their humanity will alter their present circumstances. Quite clearly, there are few, if any, grounds for this belief – not least because, as Agamben observes, '[a] permanent status of man in himself is inconceivable for the law of the nation-state' (1995: 116).[43]

The differences between the two positions can be more clearly understood by referring to the ways in which external actors, including UNRWA, have (re)interpreted their obligations and responsibilities to Palestinians. Sayigh notes that UNRWA initially encouraged refugees in Arab countries to migrate. He adds that later development projects that sought to promote 'self-reliance', including by removing of ration cards, had precisely the same aim in mind, although they were resisted by Palestinians on precisely this basis (2008: 111–12).[44] In the contemporary context, a strong Palestinian opposition has similarly emerged in response to a 'neoliberal peacebuilding' (Haddad, 2016)[45] that seeks to 'coexis[t] with the operative colonial structure instead of bringing it to a close' (Badarin, 2015: 159),[46] and which enables Israel to cooperate with Western donors and proceed apace with its colonial project (Turner, 2012; Hilal, 2015).[47] Quite clearly, a 'peace' that depoliticizes the refugee issue and excludes a history of dispossession barely deserves to be called a 'peace' at all (Haddad, 2016).[48]

UNRWA, and not the PA, is responsible for providing services to refugees. However, conditions in the camps, where there is poor infrastructure and basic services, are dire. There is also no security, as the camps are subject to extensive Israeli surveillance and imposed movement restrictions. Karim (not his real name) reiterates: 'We pay taxes for PA, but get no services because camps are the responsibility of UNRWA. [The PA] is unable to provide support.'[49]

For some refugees, the PA is part of the problem. One observes:

> The PA systemically demonizes refugee camps, and even Birzeit University graduates are treated as 4th class citizens. The PA deals with us as an epicentre of criminal acts. The political system consists of client class, business men while poverty increases…there is no middle class. After Oslo, separation has been both physical and mental. In the past camps were the center of the revolution and intellectual debate; however, now there are systematic interventions that seek to end or dissolve the refugee issue.[50]

And others blame the Arab countries.[51] Another refugee observes:

We are disappointed that the Arab countries are not doing enough to solve the refugee issue and end the occupation. The refugee issue has a regional dimension – Arab countries are responsible, but their internal issues negatively impact our cause. Arab countries allowed us to become dependent on external funding. But we will never lose hope and our rights will not be diminished by time.[52]

UNRWA's humanitarian mandate means it has a very limited ability to engage with the politics of the situation, let alone adjust and/or alter them (Hanafi, Chaaban and Seyfert, 2012: 42).[53] Indeed, in certain instances, it could even be argued to be normalizing the occupation – in one particularly egregious example, its staff constructed an emergency exit that would enable students to escape when Israel conducted military operations nearby.[54] Shadi Al Najjar,[55] a director on the board of Jalazone Volunteer Work Youth, also told me that UNRWA staff refused his request to provide protection to students during after-school training sessions.

Dissatisfaction with UNRWA is evident in refugee camps across the West Bank and Gaza Strip.[56] Given this, it is perhaps surprising that Palestinians continue to view the UN agency as an essential part of their struggle. Al Husseini observes:

However, instead of detaching the refugees from UNRWA, as most of the Western donors expected and perhaps intended, the decline in services has on the contrary increased the refugees' tendency to emphasize their political interpretation of the agency's mandate as the ultimate protector of their humanitarian and political rights. (2010: 18; also see Irfan, 2018: 81–95)[57]

This was further reiterated after proposed funding cuts caused an outcry and were denounced by Palestinian refugees as an 'international conspiracy' (Al Husseini, 2010: 18).[58] The agency was, however, in a state of crisis before this. One interviewee referred, for example, to insufficient provision (a single clinic in the camp serves 17,000 residents) and pre-pandemic medicine shortages, and claimed attested to a 'systematic effort' to reduce services.[59]

The pandemic has interfaced with these pre-existent inadequacies but has also presented its own challenges. In one illustration of the latter, Israeli settlers attacked Moussa Qattash's[60] brother with an axe during a family picnic. He received serious injuries that required surgery, but this was delayed, both because of a lack of available services and because the settlers deliberately spat on him, meaning he had to self-isolate[61] (see OCHA, 2020b).[62] Qattash also told me that he was advised to travel to Ramallah when he visited an UNRWA clinic in the camp, a proposed course of action that potentially exposed others to unacceptable risk.[63] Isolation in the confined and overcrowded camp is an ongoing challenge – when May al-Kaila, the Palestinian health minister, visited the camp on 11 July 2020 after a case upsurge, isolation spaces were the main priority for residents.[64]

The Palestinian attachment to UNRWA is at least partly due to the politicization of its work – Israel has made it clear that it wants to see the agency dissolved, which obviously influenced the Trump administration's position. And it has tried to exploit IMPACT-se's (Institute for Monitoring Peace and Cultural Tolerance in School Education) concerns about 'incitement' and anti-Semitism in UNRWA texts (IMPACT-se).[65] The Institute's report criticized supplementary materials provided to students in the pandemic, and its director even claimed that 'UNRWA-created material is, in places, more extremist than PA material it complements' (2021: 2).[66] The agency rejected these allegations and insisted that its teaching materials are regularly reviewed to ensure they are consistent with UN principles and values.[67] However, this did not satisfy the EU, which published a report that upheld these accusations and committed to reallocate funding to the PA, subject to changes in its own curriculum.[68] And the UK government cut education and healthcare funding for both the PA and UNRWA.[69]

Israel's interference in Palestinian education began when it imposed military rule following the Nakba and the establishment of the state of Israel.[70] After seizing the oPt in 1967, it used a combination of force and economic incentives[71] to ban textbooks and change and delete all national material and symbols. And, in doing so, it invoked an entirely bogus and fraudulent legitimacy. This is just one further illustration of how '[c]olonial power goes to great lengths to establish its moral and liberal narrative, as well as political supremacy' (Piterberg, 2008: 56).[72]

The pandemic in Jalazone camp

In addressing the inadequacies of the response to Covid-19 in the camp, interviewees referred to a number of different factors, including the absence of political parties and an effective national leadership. The PA was also criticized for its unclear role, focus on Ramallah and inability to execute emergency plans. Widespread scepticism about the virus and the vaccination, including the tendency to dismiss it as exaggerated or even as a political conspiracy, was attributable to a number of factors, including a lack of confidence in the PA.[73] In the first instance, we should, however, acknowledge the immense challenges involved in implementing social distancing[74] in a camp of 0.253 square kilometres with a population of around 17,000.

In June 2020, Jalazone camp became the second virus epicentre in the West Bank (after Hebron) as a result of weddings and social events, with twenty to thirty cases reported daily.[75] However, one month later the Palestinian Health Ministry claimed there were only seventy-eight confirmed cases. This could, however, have reflected a low number of tests.

Before the pandemic, camp residents had been afflicted by a number of health issues related to poor living conditions, including overcrowding, poor ventilation, inadequate sanitary facilities and the complete absence of a sewage system.[76] The pandemic interfaced with these pre-existent problems and exacerbated them. As Hilal notes, 'the coronavirus crisis exposed the absence of Palestinian sovereignty and the need to develop a new Palestinian vision and strategy' (2020: 32).[77]

UNRWA's role was initially limited to collecting data from the popular committees.[78] At the peak of the pandemic, it did not provide required services, closed clinics and began to provide packages (including a basic PPE kit and basic food items) to isolated patients only after pressure from the popular committees. Its doctors were given leave, meaning patients with chronic illnesses were left without care. In Lebanon, refugees complained that the agency only provided a minimal response to Covid-19. One refugee from the Ein El-Hilweh camp complained insufficient UNRWA funding 'left refugees dead on both sides; between health and hunger'.[79]

Samah (not her real name) contends that UNRWA's role was 'minimal' while noting that it distributed masks and sanitizers at the beginning of the pandemic. However, she adds health clinics were closed and did not provide medicine in many cases.[80] An UNRWA nurse adds the agency is unable to provide basic protective kits, like masks or sanitizers, because of a funding shortage. She observes that UNRWA services continued to operate, albeit at half of their previous capacity, and confirms that clinics were closed and medication was handed through windows.[81]

As a result, residents were obliged to meet their own health needs by establishing popular, social and voluntary committees. Local medical doctors from the camp volunteered, while other residents fundraised and launched awareness-raising campaigns about the virus and the need to disinfect the camp. One observer suggests that UNRWA support was essential for no more than one-fifth of this work.[82] This recalls the response of indigenous peoples in North America to the pandemic. Katherine Florey explains: 'Although not always beyond criticism nor enough to overcome poverty, state resistance, and other constraints, effective tribal governance has both saved lives in Indian country and provided a model of pandemic response outside it.'[83]

However, the committees have a limited ability to address the wastewater issue, which Dr Tamami claims is more dangerous than the virus. The initial impetus to establish these committees came from the Refugee Affairs Department of the PLO (which had previously sought to improve service provision by operating as an intermediary between the PA and the refugees and lobbying donors to increase UNRWA funding).[84],[85] Although the Department tried to take credit for this funding, interviewees told me it was actually raised by the popular committees. And it was only the pressure of refugees that led the PA to open the Hugo Chavez Ophthalmic Hospital,[86] which began to receive coronavirus patients in March 2020. When cases spiked in June, patients were only moved to a hotel in Ramallah (Al Bireh) and a centre in Jefna village after social media criticism of the PA. A (voluntary) medical committee was then established, whose members provided support, disinfected streets and distributed food.[87]

However, this popular mobilization was not on the scale of that shown in the First *Intifada* and there was no genuinely united national leadership to guide it. And indeed, interviewees acknowledged that some of the community initiatives at the beginning of the pandemic were short-lived[88] and also claimed that had the pandemic broken out in the First *Intifada*, a broader and more sustained public response would have been forthcoming.[89] In contrast, the organized popular committees of the First *Intifada*, which were led by political parties, successfully provided services in a number of areas, including by addressing health needs ('Towards a State of Independence', 1988: 14–21).[90]

Even when the PA responded, some of its measures were counterproductive. A lack of trust, which was compounded by the 'near-expired vaccine scandal' (see above),[91] meant residents avoided tests. Samah notes residents will only vaccinate if it is a requirement – the families of Palestinian prisoners have a clear incentive to do this, as otherwise they will not be allowed to visit Israeli prisons. One resident, whose son was first arrested at thirteen years of age and then rearrested at sixteen and a half years (he himself was arrested at the same age), was prevented from visiting his son for this reason.[92] Camp residents had an added incentive to avoid vaccination as the work permits of workers whose siblings or relatives tested positive (for the virus) were cancelled and they were banned from entering Israel for fourteen to twenty days.

The PA failed to provide information about the virus and its closures failed to acknowledge economic realities and did not provide additional support (Dalashi, interview).[93] As a result, shops in the camp remained open. Shadi Al Najjar explains:

PA lockdown affected the camp. Because there was no source of income, residents couldn't afford to stay at home. They need to work to feed their children. Many residents are banned from working in Israel for security reasons. There was no lockdown in the camp as we could not afford it. Nearby villages even used to shop in the camp during the PA lockdown.[94]

Isolation was therefore not an option for those on the economic precipice. As in other instances, the pandemic exacerbated a pre-existent vulnerability and compounded pre-existent threats to security and well-being. This is no doubt what Tabner (2020) has in mind when referring to restrictions on 'access to education, health, money, work and the maintenance of social distancing'.[95]

Vulnerability was frequently influenced by class. Sharif (2020) explains how lockdown negatively affected those who live small houses in crowded areas, and he notes the contrast with counterparts who live in spacious houses with gardens.[96] Samah observes that 'the main problem in the camp is overcrowdings and this cause the virus to spread more. The situation in the camp has gotten worse over the years and since 1949. There has been huge population growth on the same piece of land. The camp is crowded and there is disarray'.[97]

Economic factors clearly lead Palestinians to view the pandemic as a secondary consideration. Others, such as Dr Ahmad Dalahi, for example, instead claim 'the danger is more from the Israeli army and settlers'.[98] And Shadi Al Najjar argues that 'the occupation is more dangerous than the virus. People face the virus, but we have to deal with the occupation that bans everything. We are fighting the occupation while searching for our source of living and now the virus. The occupation prevents treatment and development'.[99]

Dr Abdelrahman Tamim, meanwhile, suggests that wastewater is more dangerous than the coronavirus. This untreated water, which sometimes contains Covid-19, pollutes air and water and destroys crops and agriculture when it flows into nearby villages. But UNRWA has refused to take responsibility for water treatment, and the PA has other priorities.[100] The lack of access to clean water is also affected by

Israeli policies and negligence.[101] In the Gaza Strip, the blockade and successive wars have destroyed water and sewage networks and the wastewater treatment plant (Wafi and Zaida, 2020: 12);[102] in Kufr 'Aqab, wastewater overflows in the street; and in south Hebron, residents have, as a result of land confiscation and curfews, no option but to buy – mostly contaminated – water in tanks (Human Rights Watch, 2021: 13–8; also see Abu-Sada, 2009: 427).[103]

Tamimi, in acknowledging the potential of Palestinian civil society to address this challenge, also recognizes its limitations. He observes:

> Civil Society formed a water emergency committee and initiated a water sterilization campaign. The Palestinian Environmental NGOs Network[104] cooperates with UNDP and Jerusalem Water Undertaking[105] to address water issues. But this is not enough. Palestinians are affected by wastewater from Israeli settlements located on top of hills and mountains. Wastewater and chemical material from Israeli factories in the West Bank infiltrate into the ground water and contaminate Palestinian, livestock, plants and agriculture. And Israel sells Palestinians pesticides that are prohibited by international law.[106]

Conclusion

For the inhabitants of Jalazone refugee camp, the pandemic has been one problem superimposed on top of various others. Each day, they inhabit a 'death zone' where life has little or no value. Despite UNRWA's efforts to provide assistance, conditions in the camp are 'dire' and basic human needs and requirements are not met. Residents suffer from overcrowding and poor sanitation, which make it difficult, if not impossible, to contain the virus and follow the WHO's safety guidelines. This has created unpredictable and 'death-worlds' (Mbembe, 2003: 40),[107] where residents are condemned to live a 'bare life' (Agamben, 1998: 81–6).[108] The situation looks set to deteriorate still further as declining international support decreases in the inverse proportion to growing demand for basic services.

UNRWA's ability to meet these basic needs is limited by a number of factors, including a humanitarian mandate that prevents it from addressing the challenges associated with the occupation. In the worst instances, UNRWA has been required to adapt its work to the occupation, leaving it open to the accusation of collaboration. Past historical practices that include encouraging migration and assimilation into host societies have further aggravated these suspicions.

Given this, it is perhaps surprising to note that Palestinian refugees view UNRWA as an important part of their struggle for basic human dignity. And, even more, that they view cuts to its service provision as part of an international conspiracy that ultimately seeks to remove this essential life support mechanism. This is conceivably due to a number of factors, including the politicization of the agency by the United States and Israel, and the importance of the agency as a symbolic indicator of the international community's continued commitment to Palestinian refugees.

The agency's sustainability is clearly drawn into question by the fact that it was in a state of crisis even before the Trump administration's funding cuts, and its management had been forced to consider a range of ways to save costs, including partnerships. Equally seriously, the previous US administration's renunciation of the Right of Return and general downgrading of the status of international law raises clear questions about the sustainability of the international community's commitment to uphold the Right of Return; and here it should be remembered that Israeli politicians have either refused to recognize the existence of such a right or have effectively denied its existence by making insubstantial offers in peace negotiations.

For Palestinians, the refugee issue was historically at the centre of the struggle and provided its overarching rationale and end justification. This changed after the Oslo Accords, when they became, at best, a secondary consideration. Considerably more resources have been committed, both by the PA and the 'international community' to state-building in the oPt and to security cooperation, to take two examples. Even before the pandemic, established commitments were being removed.

Camp residents are infringed on in various ways, and most notably by the political-spatial division of the oPt. The presence of a nearby settlement means that residents are reminded on a daily basis of the occupation and of the presence of the occupiers. Basic services have been eroded and life inside the camp is extremely difficult and challenging. UNRWA is clearly in no position to protect residents from the occupiers and therefore directly fails to uphold a key part of its mandate. It is therefore no surprise that Palestinians across the West Bank and Gaza Strip frequently express dissatisfaction with the agency. The concerns of Jalazone camp residents are echoed by Palestinian refugees in Lebanon.

Again, it should be reiterated that this was the case before the pandemic. However, the spread of Covid-19 exacerbated existing governance shortcomings. First, the PA is unable to operate in the camp but is actually held responsible for the inadequate response to the pandemic; similarly, low levels of vaccine uptake and the spread of mistruths and conspiracy theories reflect broader political distrust of the PA.

Second, UNRWA's role was initially limited to information collecting, despite the clear potential for the pandemic to impact on different aspects of its work, including health and education provision. And finally, both the PA and UNRWA only responded after concerted pressure by committees within the camp. However, in each instance it would clearly be inaccurate to claim the pandemic caused governance failures, as its essential 'contribution' was to highlight them in clearer detail.

Indeed, far from helping to address the pandemic, the actions of the PA and UNRWA actually threatened to exacerbate it. The PA's communications were unclear and potentially misleading, while UNRWA staff gave health advice that exposed other Palestinians to unnecessary health risks. The PA's heavy-handed implementations of closures also failed to acknowledge the very clear differences in vulnerability, and the need to take risks, between Palestinians from different socio-economic groups. Those from poorer backgrounds were more predisposed to take risks, and the public health response needed to (but did not) acknowledge and address this.

It would be too easy and simplistic to contrast the community response to the official one, and to contend that 'bottom-up' participation and community activities will sufficiently help to address and alleviate a number of the deficiencies that were shown in the official response. Both conditions in the camp and the challenges that residents face on a day-to-day basis mean that their ability to 'engage' and 'participate' are clearly limited. In addition, while a number of interviewees referred to the First *Intifada*, and their associated belief that a more effective community-based response would have been forthcoming in the late 1980s, it is essential to remember that a number of the necessary preconditions for such a response, such as an effective national leadership that is able to mobilize collective energies, are no longer in place.

Nonetheless, the response of the committees, and their role in encouraging official actors to respond to the pandemic, does offer some hope in this respect. Popular committees had also, it should be remembered, played a role in helping to generate funding for UNRWA and health provision in the camp. If it is unrealistic to expect the committees to take a leading role in responding to future responses to future public health emergencies, it is perhaps more realistic to expect they will function as part of networks that seek to produce a more effective and timely official response. In addition, it could also be considered if the committees and other public associations could function as responses that official actors could draw upon and utilize. The case of Jalazone also demonstrates that the root cause of the refugee issue needs to be addressed at a political level. This includes granting their right of return on the basis of established UN resolutions.

Conclusion

In the pandemic, respect for human life, and more precisely the lives of the colonized, has further degraded from an already low point. The essential principle that some lives are worth more than others and that some are more disposable, which was always implicitly understood, is now explicitly articulated, to the point where it has become unavoidable. In this 'necroeconomy', lives are rendered and disposed of without a second thought. Unvaccinated Palestinian workers and prisoners, the dumping of infected workers at checkpoints and the trading of near-expired vaccines for political benefit/s all speak of not just a disregard but an open contempt for the value of human life.

While speaking to interviewees, I was struck by the fact that they did not view the pandemic as a priority that should be privileged over other challenges. They saw the difficult economic situation, settler attacks and Israeli eviction policies as more pressing priorities. Especially in the case of the Gaza Strip, they frequently emphasized the pandemic was low on their list of priorities or did not even feature on it at all. From my perspective, I found it more useful to view the pandemic response through the prism of colonial power and to understand its deficiencies and shortcomings as an outgrowth of pre-established issues and problems. The inadequacies of the PA's response, Israel's actions/inactions and the difficulties of collective mobilization under established conditions all became much clearer when viewed and understood from this (colonial) perspective. This reality is of course denied by key international actors, Israel and, perhaps most significantly of all, the PA. It is to this extent wholly deficient to understand and engage this as a public health challenge or issue, as this insufficiently acknowledges the centrality of underlying political dynamics and relations.

Aspects of the pandemic response cannot be understood in isolation but only in relation to other aspects or dimensions of the contemporary

Palestinian situation. For example, the inability of Palestinians to effectively organize in response to the pandemic should be viewed as a symptom of the disruptions of Palestinian social and political life by colonial power. Fragmentation of land and population has made organization more difficult, and so has the establishment of the PA, which has more often than not sought to co-opt, rather than enable and develop, public energies. Similarly, the PA's declaration of a state emergency has more clearly enabled the expansion of executive power/s than the emergence of an effective public health strategy or framework.

Far from viewing public participation as a potential resource that can be applied, the PA has more frequently seen it as a possible threat to its established privileges and entitlements. In any case, it is important to recognize that under radically altered objective realities (i.e. the difference between the First *Intifada* and the current situation), the potential of public participation to effectively respond to public needs and requirements is substantially limited. In Jalazone refugee camp, for example, popular, social and voluntary committees responded to shortcomings in UNRWA provision by engaging in awareness-raising and fundraising activities. However, interviewees in the refugee camp suggested these activities were relatively short-lived and in any case were not on the scale of the popular mobilization that occurred during the First *Intifada*. In any case, it is quite clear that 'participation' and 'public engagement' cannot be spoken of as panaceas that offer a solution to every shortcoming and deficit of Palestinian public life.

The politicization of the PA's pandemic response was another frequently mentioned concern. In the case of Palestine, this term refers to the role of the PA and, by extended implication, the marginalization of civil society and the gap between the rulers and the ruled. The PA showed a rare initiative and purpose in initially responding to the pandemic, but it was unable to sustain this over time and ultimately lapsed back into established patterns and tendencies, as the vaccine scandal so clearly demonstrated. The absence of a pandemic plan was a clear weakness that acted to the detriment of an effective public health response.

Over time, it appears that the PA's public health measures became increasingly fatigued and that, both as a result of a lack of will and resources, it was unable to protect public health. This was also the case in the Strip, where effective measures introduced helped to ensure that no cases were recorded in the initial seven months of the pandemic (although here remember that the Strip was already largely cut off from the outside world and potential sources of infection). However, in contrast to the West Bank, where preventative measures gradually lost impetus and focus, Hamas's weakening of lockdown measures instead appeared to be a response to public pressure. In the absence of democratic means of expression and growing public discontent that in the view of some interviewees potentially jeopardized its rule, it had a clear incentive to make concessions of this kind.

The vaccine scandal did not merely undermine (already low) public confidence in the PA, but it also harmed public health measures, including by giving renewed impetus to fear-mongering and ill-informed scepticism about the (completely safe) vaccine. The scandal was also of interest because it again reiterated the PA's failure to acknowledge, let alone challenge, the (neo) colonial conditions under which it is obliged to engage with the Israeli enemy and also the international community more generally. Even more seriously, it again reiterated the PA's willingness to engage on these terms and to accept the (grossly unequal and unfair) concessions that it has been granted. Furthermore, as in the case of Israel's siege of the Strip, it has actually encouraged the colonial aggressor to strengthen its grip. In continually demonstrating a willingness to negotiate from a condition of weakness, the PA can of course hardly complain when it is regarded and treated with the contempt it so richly deserves.

And it is of course similarly deficient to expect the PA to acknowledge or challenge the existing status quo when it is effectively an outgrowth of it – to be more precise, its effective role is to uphold and perpetuate (neo) colonial arrangements rather than challenge or undermine them. Indeed, recent revelations suggest that under the guise of security coordination and the benign interventions of the 'international community', the PA has come dangerously close to effectively collaborating with the colonial power. Despite this, there is little sign of cooperation during the pandemic in Hebron, when the H1/H2 divide continued to impede the – disconnected and small scale – efforts of the PA police to take preventative actions. However, it must be understood what is required at this stage is not an acceptance of this 'colonial' case, but rather a *reversion* to what was previously an accepted framework of reference and consensus within the PLO. To the same extent, political opinion needs to follow the lead of academic research, which has increasingly converged on the colonial features and attributes of the contemporary situation in the oPt.

The PA's decision to distribute vaccines to senior PA officials and their families was also highly controversial.[1] Interviewees in Hebron also cited Fatah's dominance of the emergency committees as a factor that undermined public confidence and the emergence and development of an effective public health response. Its prioritization of Ramallah and failure to focus on Hebron – which at one stage accounted for more than two-thirds of Covid-19 cases in the West Bank – was a further source of grievance – however, here it should again be stressed that these resentments can be traced back to pre-pandemic governance trends in the West Bank.

In the Gaza Strip, interviewees cited growing corruption among Hamas officials as a contributor to non-compliance with lockdown measures – this is an interesting development because a large part of Hamas's historical appeal rested on the fact that it was seen as more honest and transparent than Fatah. Lack of trust in public representatives and institutions has clear implications for public willingness to accept and uphold public health guidelines. In this and numerous other respects, the pandemic is deeply political.

In the pandemic, public relations, or the need to be seen to be taking effective action, quickly emerged as an important aspect of the government response. The need to take control of the 'narrative' and give the impression of an effective and comprehensive response became a priority for governments across the world. In Palestine, some interviewees expressed concern that this had actually emerged as the preponderant priority. This was suggested by some Hebron interviewees, who claimed that PA public health measures were 'for show' and were primarily intended to create the impression that something was being done. In reality, the response in Hebron appears to be uncoordinated, with interviewees claiming that public health measures were either limited or non-existent. Interviewees in the South Hebron Hills also claimed that the PA's main concern and priority was to be seen to be acting, rather than actually providing an effective and comprehensive public health response.

Interviewees also frequently referred to the continuity between the pre-pandemic and pandemic phases. This was noted in relation to colonialism, but also with reference to the PA's governance. To this extent, the virus ruthlessly exploited existing gaps in the Palestinian health system that left Palestinians exposed and vulnerable. Similarly, in the Gaza Strip, Hamas's distribution of funding to Hamas hospitals and clinics meant that the – depleted and beleaguered – health service functioned on the basis of political loyalty rather than efficiency and/ or public needs. The pandemic also served to further underline and reiterate pre-existing shortcomings and weaknesses within the health system that can be traced back to the pre-Oslo period, when Israel routinely failed to meet obligations established by international law. Similarly, in the Gaza Strip, severely depleted health resources, an inability to access clean water and one of the most densely populated territories in the world created a perfect incubating environment for Covid-19. This was also the case in Kufr 'Aqab, where long-term Israeli neglect left residents exposed to the virus.

Israel's heralded status as a global vaccine 'leader' therefore conceals a grossly unjust status quo in which the public health disparity between Palestinians and Israelis has become another dimension of the apartheid reality. The Israeli government has not just consistently denied its public health obligations to Palestinians, but has gone to great lengths to frustrate an effective Palestinian response, both through direct intervention and inaction. For example, it has both failed to ensure equitable vaccine distribution or acknowledge obligations established under international law, and has also destroyed Covid-19 testing centres and attacked Palestinian hospitals and health facilities. However, it did seek to 'securitize' Palestinian non-compliance and present it as a 'threat' to Israel's sanctity and well-being. However, this occludes the essential fact that Palestinians will die both as a result of Israel's callous and inhuman disregard, and as a result of its wilful intent.

Israel has simultaneously evidenced a disinterest in Palestinians' health and well-being and an interest in extracting as much political capital from the situation as possible. In precisely these terms, Fanon had, in referring to the colonizer, spoken of 'an almost mechanical sense of detachment and mistrust of even the things that are most positive and most profitable to the population' (1994: 139).[2] While it has been intermittently interested and disinterested, engaged and disengaged, Israel has never offered the pretence of being concerned with Palestinians or Palestinian public health, and this, while being consistent with its established colonial rule, clearly distinguishes it from historical examples of colonialism. Indeed, this has applied to the extent that it has failed to take actions that could conceivably protect and uphold its own public health measures. Quite clearly, the Palestinian case also does not align with Foucault's presentation of 'health' interventions as a continually expanding spectrum of control, surveillance and supervision.

Quite clearly, the very premise of conflict resolution is negated from the outset by Israel's steadfast refusal to recognize the history of the 'conflict' or the fundamental injustice that has been inflicted on Palestinians. Wolfe has previously spoken of a 'logic of elimination that is not invariably genocidal' (2006: 388),[3] and this perfectly captures an Israeli rejectionism that can be traced back to *terra nullius* and chased into the dark realms of Zionist ideology. Israel wills, as Rabin made clear in the case of the Gaza Strip, the disappearance but cannot fully realize this aspiration without violating the sacrosanct international prohibition of genocide. In its absence, 'transfer' still remains a tantalizing possibility that is openly discussed in mainstream Israeli politics. However, it is not just sufficient that Palestinians are not seen; rather, they must disappear to the greatest extent possible. Whereas previous generations of Israeli politicians merely contented themselves with ignoring Palestinians (as in Golda Meir's infamous formulation), their successors go to every length possible to ensure that the Palestinian aspiration to political significance is pre-emptively denied and negated.

During the pandemic, Israel has also continued with dispossessions, forced evictions and military operations, despite the potential for such actions to imperil Palestinian health and well-being. As in other instances, inaction has been accompanied by deliberate actions that have the clear potential to further inflame and exacerbate the pandemic. In Hebron, this has allegedly extended to Israeli settlers actively seeking to encourage virus spread (by, for example, spitting on door handles or causing deliberate disruption). As would be expected in a city where the settlers are effectively in control and settlers serve in the Israeli army, similar allegations have been made against Israeli soldiers. In such instances, Israel does not just disrupt but actively enables the spread of the virus. As Sitta notes, this is consistent with Israel's past efforts to cultivate a typhoid epidemic for its own political purposes.[4]

This analysis of Israel's actions can and must extend to the role of international organizations and actors, who have singularly failed to make Israel comply with its fundamental international obligations and responsibilities. This is of course by no means unique to the pandemic, as Israel's contempt for international opinion and flagrant disregard was already well-established, to the point of not even needing to be acknowledged and/or reiterated. Palestinians had the unique misfortunate to suffer the Trump administration's disingenuous and fraudulent 'peace' initiative at the same time as the pandemic, with the consequence that one national dislocation and tragedy was superimposed on top of another. Even the PA found itself in a position where it could no longer uphold proposed terms that were effectively a surrender that denied Palestinian national (i.e. political) aspirations. Any sustainable critique must also extend to the peace process itself, which must be viewed and treated as a mechanism of colonial power rather than as a means through which a non-existent 'conflict' can be resolved upon the basis of mutually acceptable propositions.

In looking to the future in Palestine, we should not therefore speak of the 'post-pandemic' stage as if it is an entirely novel stage; rather, we should instead see it as the intensification of pre-existing tendencies, patterns and relations. In this regard, it is instructive to refer to Judith Butler's allusion to 'forms of "radical inequality, nationalism, and capitalist exploitation" [that have found] "ways to reproduce and strengthen themselves within the pandemic zones"'.[5] The pandemic should therefore not be viewed in isolation but should instead be understood in the context of, and to a substantial degree as an extension of, a global imperial context that continues to perpetuate inequality and exploitation.

While the challenges that confront Palestinians in the aftermath of the pandemic have been 'scaled up' (often to exaggerated and otherwise grossly distorted proportions), they are not fundamentally different from those that presented themselves in the pre-pandemic period. Similarly, the fundamental adjustments that are required are essentially the same as those that were needed before the pandemic.

For outside observers accustomed to the entitlements, guarantees and securities of life in the developed world, the pandemic has brought death uncomfortably close and exposed its inhabitants to the same risks and threats as their 'undeveloped' counterparts. To some extent, the virus was something of an equalizer, in that it threatened the 'developed' and 'undeveloped' alike, and this was confirmed by crude and somewhat rudimentary preventative measures and high death tolls in the 'developed' world. However, in the aftermath of the pandemic, this has now changed, as global inequalities and injustices have again reasserted and imposed themselves.

However, this overlooks the fact that the pandemic was not regarded in the same terms by Western and Palestinian audiences. In large part, this is attributable to the fact that Palestinians are more accustomed to death, to the point where it is viewed as part of everyday life rather than simply as its termination or end point. In the Gaza Strip, for example, it was noticeable that inhabitants regarded the virus with a degree of fatalism and resignation, while in Jalazone refugee camp it was seen as a secondary consideration that was subordinate to the issue of wastewater disposal. In the first instance, death is accepted or even willed, whereas in the second it is seen as likely to emanate from any number of possible sources. Both serve to again reiterate the essential point that the pandemic was by no means exceptional or to be regarded as an abrupt departure from 'business-as-usual'.

In other words, the pandemic by no means inaugurated a 'state of exception' – rather, it instead appeared as the perpetuation of a persistent condition of insecurity in which Palestinian lives were reduced and degraded and a sense of hopelessness was perpetuated and ingrained. The pandemic was not, to this extent, viewed as a justification for the introduction of different measures and intervention but was instead, for many Palestinians, regarded as an inconvenience that needed to be worked around.

On one level, I found this comforting, as it served as a further reiteration of the Palestinian determination to persevere in the face of innumerable challenges. The toughness and resilience that has steered Palestinians through innumerable national catastrophes, therefore, remains intact and perseveres. However, from a different perspective, I could see that this 'resilience' instead originated in a failure to acknowledge the seriousness of the pandemic and its potential to kill and inflict lasting harm. For instance, in Kufr 'Aqab, Palestinians from other 'locked down' areas of the West Bank visited to attend wedding and parties, despite the substantial health risks this posed to others, and the vulnerable in particular. Clearly, they did not fully grasp the extent of the risks they were taking, with both their own health and the health of others. While it is certainly the case that, as in the case of Jalazone refugee camp, the mixed messages of the PA can be criticized, at some point individuals have to take responsibility for their own actions and consider those around them. However, I was also aware that Palestinians often had no choice to take these risks, irrespective of their knowledge of the virus. Their actions were not willed, and therefore indicative of this fabled 'resilience' but were instead compelled, for the reason that it was impossible for them to otherwise sustain themselves and their families.

From this perspective, the Palestinian response did not appear as pragmatic or even brave, but instead appeared to be an outgrowth of fatalism or a resignation to the course of ongoing events. While it is relatively easy to see how this could be conflated with, or even mistaken for, 'resilience', their effects are quite clearly different – to this extent, 'resilience' produces an ability to persevere in the face of setbacks and to withstand formidable blows; 'fatalism', in contrast, inculcates a passivity and appears almost as a defence mechanism, which functions to protect the holder from the insight that they have no ability to alter, or even effect, the world around them. Fatalism turns the individual in on themselves, producing a passive introspection that effectively turns them away from the world outside.

Here Ghanim's (2008) concept of thanatopolitics is particularly invaluable as it clarifies that it is the threat of death, rather than death itself, that is utilized and made to function in the service of political designs. Israel has long recognized the utility of uncertainty as a political device, and has come to appreciate and understand that the threatened imposition of a measure, whether a visa requirement or military force, can be effective as its actual implementation. This was clearly illustrated by the case study of Kufr 'Aqab, which explained how residents live in a perpetual state of uncertainty and flux, which has been deliberately cultivated and exploited by the Israeli authorities. In referring to this reality, one resident observed that they 'lived here to wait', again reiterating that their future was not in their own hands and that the course of their own lives would be decided by others.

Quite clearly, and here Memmi, Fanon and Foucault are important reference points, a system of repression is only fully realized and effective at the point when it is internalized by the colonized, for precisely the reason that it offsets the need for the colonizer to apply repressive measures. This is a perverse and grotesque of a pedagogical process in which the colonized 'learn' appropriate conducts and forms of deportment.

I therefore viewed these attitudes and decisions as less of an affirmation of Palestinian 'resistance' and more of a submission to a necro-political arrangement that obliges Palestinians to accept a subsistence existence at the cost of their own health and well-being. The terms of this transaction are not paid in hard currency, but rather by their own lives and their right to a meaningful and secure existence. It is not merely that Palestinians are lost in the course of a struggle for political recognition, but rather that their lives are required to sustain and perpetuate this necropolitics, whose implications are implicitly familiar but whose significance is rarely, if ever, acknowledged by those who enable and perpetuate it. This, I would suggest, is the most important insight that can be extracted from the pandemic: in the Palestinian territories, 'life' became meaningless for the reason that death long ago became the price that many Palestinians pay for a futile and violent existence that hardly approximates to 'life' in any meaningful sense of the word. For Gazans, it is the struggle for dignity, freedom and justice, and not the pandemic, that is the key priority. In the wretched Gaza Strip, the sealed-off Kufr 'Aqab or the desperate environs of Jalazone refugee camp, 'life' is a living death in which surplus and unwanted 'populations' are consigned and corralled to suffer their fate.

In confronting a dire situation, Palestinians continue to resist colonization and dispossession. Residents of Kufr 'Aqab who insist on keeping their Jerusalem IDs despite the various challenges and privations they endure as a result are just one example among innumerable others. The virus has also to some extent unified Palestinians in historical Palestine who experience the ongoing reality of fragmentation, as was shown by a general strike of 18 May 2021 that broke out in response to an appeal from a Palestinian citizen of Israel. Even Kufr 'Aqab, which otherwise remained open during the pandemic, observed the strike by shutting down for a day – in this and other instances and respects, resistance emerged as a foremost priority for Palestinians in the pandemic.

Interviewees

Gaza Strip

Yara (not her real name) – an activist and resident of Gaza. WhatsApp conversation 28 May 2021.

Dr Yehia Abed, Yehia Abed MD, MPH, Dr. PH, Al Quds University, School of Public Health, Gaza City, Gaza, WhatsApp conversation, 11 May 2021.

Interview, director of training and scientific research department at Gaza Community Mental Health Programme – GCMHP, Messenger conversation, 5 May 2021.

Amjad Yaghi, a young freelance journalist in Gaza. Zoom interview. 10 June 2021.

Ahmad, not his real name, in the field of nursing and psychology, Gaza. Messenger conversation, 3 May 2021.

Lina, not her real name, health professional and researcher, Messenger conversation, 2 May 2021.

Saleh Abu Shamala, Youth Policy Club coordinator and researcher at Civitas Institute, Zoom meeting, 5 June 2021.

Mohamed Ramadan, Monitoring and Evaluation Consultant, UNFPA (United Nations Fund for Population Activities).

Hebron

Dr Hazem Ashhab, MD, head of Gastroenterology,·Al-Ahli Hospital. Member of National Committee for CORONA. Zoom interview, 11 June 2021.

Hisham Sharabati was an activist in the First *Intifada*. He currently coordinates the Hebron Defense Committee. Messenger conversation, 9 October 2020.

Elias al-Arja, chairman of the Arab Hotel Association. He is general manager of the Bethlehem Hotel in Bethlehem, the Nativity Hotel in Beit Jala and the Angel Hotel in Beit Jala.

Fawaz Abu Aisheh, employee at the Municipality of Hebron, Messenger conversation, 15 June 2021.

Manal (not her real name), resident of Tel Remeida, Messenger conversation.

Nour Abu Aisha, merchant, Messenger conversation, 13 June 2021.

Fuad al-Amour, activist and coordinator of the Protection and Sumud Committee, who works in the Mountains of Southern Hill in South Hebron Hills and Massafir Yatta. Messenger interview, 7 July 2021.

Shireen Abu Akleh, journalist at Al Jazeera TV. Telephone conversation, 25 June 2021. Shireen was killed on 11 May 2022 by an Israeli sniper while reporting in the city of Jenin.

Majed, not his real name, media person. Messenger conversation, 24 June 2021.

Salwa Najjab, MD, is a specialist in obstetrics, gynaecology and gynaecological cytology. She is a senior technical advisor at Juzoor Foundation Health and Social Development. She is a member of the independent fact-finding committee on the Pfizer vaccine. She co-founded a number of influential grassroots Palestinian organizations. She is also a member of the MENA Health Policy Forum, the Palestinian Health Policy Forum and the World Bank Civil Society Consultative Group for Health, Nutrition and Population. Personal interview, Exeter, UK, 4 September 2021.

Manal (not her real name), a resident of Tel Remeida, Messenger conversation, 22 December 2021.

Kufr ʿAqab

Khalid (not his real name), a Kufr ʿAqab resident, Jerusalem ID married to West Bank ID, WhatsApp conversation, 16 August 2021.

Rula (not her real name), pharmacist and researcher, 3 August 2021 Zoom interview.

Jamal Jumaʾ, coordinator of Palestinian Anti-Apartheid Wall grassroots campaign. Zoom interview, 15 August 2021.

Munir Zughayer, an activist, chairperson of the local neighbourhood committees of north Jerusalem. WhatsApp conversation, 5 August 2021.

Ola Awad-Shakhshir, minister of Palestinian Central Bureau of Statistics, Zoom interview, 16 December 2021.

Salma (not her real name), a housewife and resident of Kufr 'Aqab. She
has a West Bank ID and her husband and children have Jerusalem IDs.
WhatsApp conversation, 9 August 2021.

Mona (not her real name), a housewife and resident of Kufr 'Aqab. She holds
a Jerusalem ID, and her husband and children holding West Bank IDs,
6 August 2021, WhatsApp conversation.

Ibrahim (not his real name), a Kufr 'Aqab resident and West Bank ID holder
who is married to a Jerusalem ID holder, Messenger conversation, 10-08-
2021.

Jalazone

Dina (not her real name), a nurse who lives in Jalazone, Zoom interview,
15 December 2021.

Layla (not her real name), a kindergarten teacher who lives in Jalazone, Zoom
interview, 3 January 2022.

Ahmad Dalashi, internal medicine doctor at Ramallah Hospital and the
medical chief of the coronavirus emergency committee in Jalazone Camp.
Zoom interview, 30 January 2022.

Karim (not his real name), a resident of Jalazone, 5 September 2020,
Telephone conversation.

Shadi Al Najjar, a member of Board of Directors, Jalazone Volunteer Work
Youth. Zoom interview, 7 January 2021.

Moussa Qattash, a member of Jalazone Volunteer Work Youth. Zoom
interview, 7 January 2021.

Samah, not her real name, a kindergarten teacher at the Young Women's
Christian Association who lives in Jalazone, Zoom interview, 3 January
2022.

Dr Abdelrahman Tamimi, assistant professor of strategic planning and future
studies at the Arab American University. An expert in the field of water
resources. Zoom interview, 27 April 2022.

Notes

Introduction

1 The Palestinian Authority was created by the Oslo Accords. Along with security coordination, it is all that remains of the 1993 agreement. After Hamas seized the Gaza Strip in 10–15 June 2007, Oslo II only applied to the West Bank. It divided the West Bank into three areas, A, B and C, that each operates under different administrative rules. Area A is administered by the PA and only accounts for 4 per cent of the occupied West Bank; Area B is jointly administered by Israel and the PA, and accounts for 25 per cent; Area C, which is fully controlled by Israel and includes the settlements, accounts for 69 per cent. Palestinian access to Jerusalem is controlled by a permit system. After Hamas seized the Gaza Strip on 10–15 June 2007, it was completely severed from the West Bank. The Hebron Protocol, which was signed on 15 January 1997, divides Hebron city into H-1 (under PA) and H-2 (under Israeli military control) (JPS, 1997: 131). The South Hebron Hills are part of Area C.

2 Quran, Fadi and Mustafa, TaHani (2020). Palestine and COVID-19: Lessons for Leadership during Times of Crisis. Al Shabaka, 09 October. https://al-shabaka.org/commentaries/palestine-and-covid-19-lessons-for -leadership-during-times-of-crisis/ (accessed 11 June 2021).

3 OCHA (2020). State of Emergency: Palestine's COVID-19 Response Plan, 26 March. https://reliefweb.int/report/occupied-palestinian -territory/state-emergency-palestine-s-covid-19-response-plan (accessed 10 June 2021).

4 Elias al-Arja, chairman of the Arab Hotel Association. He is the general manager of the Bethlehem Hotel in Bethlehem, the Nativity Hotel in Beit Jala and the Angel Hotel in Beit Jala.
    WhatsApp conversation. 22 February 2021.

5 Salwa Najjab, follow-up interview, FaceTime conversation 18 August 2022.

6 World Health Organization (WHO) (2022). World Health Day 2022 – Strengthening Health Systems and Empowering Communities,

7 April. http://www.emro.who.int/opt/news/world-health-day-2022
-strengthening-health-systems-and-empowering-communities.html
(accessed 27 June 2021).

7 Gollom, Mark (2021). Why Israel is Leading the World with COVID-19
Vaccinations. *CBC News*, 02 January. https://www.cbc.ca/news/world
/israel-covid-vaccinations-1.5859396?fbclid=IwAR0m0laVvHbW2
acbdzPRmJIhRuyIBoDa6JENiZZz1qe2QFLuQmjxAKNmii4 (accessed
23 April 2021).

8 El Haroun, Zaineh (2021). Palestinian Hospitals Fill Up as Israel Loosens
COVID-19 Restrictions. *Reuters*, 09 March. https://www.reuters.com
/article/us-health-coronavirus-israel-palestinian/palestinian-hospitals
-fill-up-as-israel-loosens-covid-19-restrictions-idUSKBN2B128P?il=0
&fbclid=IwAR1ROQQz_Wf-yEFPS_lCGddvdXAZgGfwE0Eo-qsSw
-6kcRX2paG0eWuQ8D0 (accessed 23 April 2021).

9 Medical Aid for Palestinians (MAP) (2022). Coronavirus Situation
Updates, 9 February. https://www.map.org.uk/about-map/map
-coronavirus-situation-updates (accessed 03 March 2022).

10 Medical Aid for Palestinians (MAP) (2021). Open Letter to the
University of Oxford: 'Our World in Data' Misrepresents Israel's
Vaccination Rates, 22 April. https://www.map.org.uk/news/archive/
post/1221-open-letter-to-the-university-of-oxford-our-world-in-data
-misrepresents-israelas-vaccination-rates?fbclid=IwAR3PmEA6XfktE
Mk3jx6-WGPiKcMZ38x3nwXCxdSMHiSDwxgkjW7XsMAxsMM
(accessed 02 May 2021).

11 Independent (2021). Israel Rebuffs WHO Vaccine Request for Palestinian
Medics, amid OUTCRY over Disparity, 08 January. https://www
.independent.co.uk/news/world/middle-east/israel-palestine-coronavirus
-vaccine-b1784474.html?fbclid=IwAR2Sut7ykl7PAw1W4y66sBjedlhRt
WgfkeWjLPqkMDs-sbXBWkoPmUxnbMQ (accessed 02 May 2021).

12 Rapoport, Meron (2021). Israel Denies COVID Vaccine to Palestinian
Student at Tel Aviv University. +972 Magazine, 03 March. https://www
.972mag.com/palestinian-student-covid-tau/ (accessed 02 May 2021).

13 Amnesty International, UK (2021). Israel: Denying Covid-19 Vaccine
to Palestinians is 'institutionalised discrimination', 6 January. https://
www.amnesty.org.uk/press-releases/israel-denying-covid-19-vaccine
-palestinians-institutionalised-discrimination (accessed 14 May 2021).

14 Lazaroff, Tovah (2021). Israel Debates Banning COVID-19 Vaccines for Gaza Until Captives Released. *The Jerusalem Post*, 15 February. https://www.jpost.com/arab-israeli-conflict/israel-debates-linking-covid-19-vaccines-for-gaza-with-captive-release-659066 (accessed 14 May 2021).

15 Gisha-Legal Center for Freedom of Movement (2021). Gisha and 29 Other Israeli, Palestinian and International Health and Human Rights Organizations: Israel must Provide Necessary Vaccines to Palestinians, 06 January.

16 Anton, G. (2008). Blind Modernism and Zionist Waterscape The Huleh Drainage Project. *Jerusalem Quarterly* 35: 90.

17 Garbett, Lucy (2020). Palestinian Workers in Israel Caught between Indispensable and Disposable. Middle East Research and Information Project (MERIP), 15 May. https://merip.org/2020/05/palestinian-workers-in-israel-caught-between-indispensable-and-disposable/ (accessed 13 May 2021).

18 Rasgon, Adam (2021). After Harsh Criticism, Israel Says it will Vaccinate Palestinians Who Hold Work Permits. *The New York Times*, 28 February. https://www.nytimes.com/2021/02/28/world/israel-vaccine-palestine.html?fbclid=IwAR09glRE2lKGmW2uUnp-50df1muvk3MLUFtmL4jKHE9ZPaeBfPonUBh6kik (accessed 16 May 2021).

19 The Times of Israel (2021). Vaccination Drive for Palestinian Workers Delayed Amid Reported Budget Dispute, 06 March. https://www.timesofisrael.com/vaccination-drive-for-palestinian-workers-delayed-amid-reported-budget-dispute/ (accessed 16 May 2021).

20 Al-Jazeera (2021). Israel Starts Vaccinating Palestinian Workers after Delays, 08 March. https://www.aljazeera.com/news/2021/3/8/israel-starts-vaccinating-palestinian-workers-after-delays (accessed 16 May 2021).

21 Interestingly, when I spoke to one Palestinian activist from the First *Intifada*, he claimed this would not have happened then – see Naser-Najjab, N. (2020). Palestinian Leadership and the Contemporary Significance of the First Intifada. *Race & Class* 62(2): 61–79.

22 Al Waara, Akram (2020). 'They dumped him like trash': Palestinian with Suspected Coronavirus Symptoms Thrown Out of Israel. Middle East Eye, 23 March. https://www.middleeasteye.net/news/coronavirus-palestine-labourer-found-near-west-bank-checkpoint-covid19 (accessed 09 February 2021).

23 Stub, Zev (2021). Palestinian Labor Limited due to Corona, Israeli Builders Struggling. *The Jerusalem Post*, 07 January. https://www.jpost .com/israel-news/palestinian-labor-limited-due-to-corona-israeli -builders-struggling-654614 (accessed 16 October 2021).

24 Abu Al Hayat, Maya (2021). Israel Holds All the Cards in the West Bank – It should Vaccinate Everyone. *The Guardian*, 31 January. https:// www.theguardian.com/commentisfree/2021/jan/31/israel-west-bank -vaccinate-palestinians?fbclid=IwAR0dZIXhbiz9eA9lN-8jHBK07dBRO s0SYP1DkCPLOyCbHGpQO8nB2ucBGCI.

25 Stub, Zev (2021). Palestinian Labor Limited due to Corona, Israeli Builders Struggling. *The Jerusalem Post*, 07 January. https://www.jpost .com/israel-news/palestinian-labor-limited-due-to-corona-israeli -builders-struggling-654614 (accessed 11 September 2021).

26 Berda, Yael (2017). *Living Emergency: Israel's Permit Regime in the Occupied West Bank*. Redwood City: Stanford University Press.

27 Hanieh, A. and Ziadah, R. (2022). Pandemic Effects: COVID-19 and the Crisis of Development in the Middle East. *Development and Change* 53(6): 1308–34.

28 Maltz, Judy (2021). Israel to Send Thousands of Vaccines to Countries Opening Embassies in Jerusalem. *Haaretz*, 23 February. https://www .haaretz.com/israel-news/israel-to-transfer-symbolic-amount-of-covid -vaccines-to-palestinians-1.9562653?fbclid=IwAR2S9o19JGp3ULPNY t2NC0D7kpcqeW3Z-8M4uWUQ7ovsaV8X05GlIt_snQ0 (accessed 02 May 2021).

29 Maltz, Judy (2021). Israel to Send Thousands of Vaccines to Countries Opening Embassies in Jerusalem. *Haaretz*, 23 February. https://www .haaretz.com/israel-news/israel-to-transfer-symbolic-amount-of-covid -vaccines-to-palestinians-1.9562653?fbclid=IwAR2S9o19JGp3ULPNY t2NC0D7kpcqeW3Z-8M4uWUQ7ovsaV8X05GlIt_snQ0 (accessed 02 May 2021).

30 Al-Jazeera (2021). Thousands of Palestinians attend Friday Prayers at al-Aqsa Mosque, 16 April. https://www.aljazeera.com/news/2021/4/16 /palestinians-hold-aqsa-prayers-in-largest-gathering-since-covid19 (accessed 23 May 2020).

31 The Palestine Information Center (2020). Sheikh Omar al-Kiswani Warns Against Recent Israeli Surveying of Aqsa Mosque. The Palestinian

Information Center. 15 January. https://english.palinfo.com/news/2021/1/15/Sheikh-Kiswani-warns-against-recent-Israeli-surveying-of-Aqsa-Mosque (accessed 23 December 2020).

32 B'Tselem (2020). The Israeli Information Center for Human Rights in the Occupied Territories. Hagai El-Ad's address at the European Parliament Committee on Human Rights, 16 November. https://www.btselem.org/facing_expulsion_blog/20201116_european_parliament_committee_on_human_rights_address (accessed 16 January 2021).

33 Hasson, Nir (2020). Israel Shuts Palestinian Coronavirus Testing Clinic in East Jerusalem. *Haaretz*, 15 April. https://www.haaretz.com/israel-news/.premium-israeli-police-raid-palestinian-coronavirus-testing-clinic-in-east-jerusalem-1.8767788 (accessed 02 June 2020).

34 WAFA News Agency (2021). Ramallah Office of a Health Group Raided by Israeli Occupation Forces, Ransacked and Hard Discs Seized, 08 March. https://english.wafa.ps/Pages/Details/123580 (accessed 15 September 2021).

35 Levy, Gideon and Levak, Alex (2021). It's Not the First Time a Palestinian Dies This Way During a Nighttime Israeli Army Raid. *Haaretz*, 11 March. https://www.haaretz.com/israel-news/.premium.MAGAZINE-it-s-not-the-first-time-a-palestinian-dies-this-way-during-a-nighttime-idf-raid-1.9613030?fbclid=IwAR3sSNny6ZIi0CFVdTd7xriQB0XCMXRAmma_G-7HPDkwpm3PSduiXhXi7vA (accessed 11 June 2021).

36 Sa'di, A. H. (2016). *Thorough Surveillance: The Genesis of Israeli Policies of Population Management, Surveillance and Political Control towards the Palestinian Minority*. Manchester: Manchester University Press.

37 The Palestine Chronicle (2021). Israeli Forces Demolish Palestinian Village for 183rd Time, 17 February. https://www.palestinechronicle.com/israeli-forces-demolish-palestinian-village-for-183rd-time/ (accessed 16 May 2021).

38 OCHA (2020). COVID-19 Emergency Situation Report 18 (9–22 September 2020), 22 September. https://www.ochaopt.org/content/covid-19-emergency-situation-report-18 (accessed 08 January 2021).

39 B'Tselem (2020). The Israeli Information Center for Human Rights in the Occupied Territories. In Pandemic, of all Times: Number of Palestinians Israel has Left Homeless Hits Four-Year Record, 02 November. https://www.btselem.org/press_releases/20201104_number_of_palestinians

_israel_left_homeless_hits_four_year_record_in_pandemic (accessed 14 December 2020).

40 B'Tselem (2021). The Israeli Information Center for Human Rights in the Occupied Territories. A Regime of Jewish Supremacy from the Jordan River to the Mediterranean Sea: This is Apartheid, 12 January. https://www.btselem.org/publications/fulltext/202101_this_is_apartheid (accessed 03 May 2021).

41 Nasser, Tamara (2020). Court Denies Palestinian Prisoners Right to COVID-19 Protection. The Electronic Intifada, 27 July. https://electronicintifada.net/blogs/tamara-nassar/court-denies-palestinian-prisoners-right-covid-19-protection (accessed 12 January 2021).

42 Adalah (2020). The Legal Center for Arab Minority Rights. Israeli Supreme Court Rules: Palestinian Prisoners have no Right to Social Distancing Protection against COVID-19, 23 July. https://www.adalah.org/en/content/view/10063 (accessed 23 November 2020).

43 Melhem, Ahmad (2021). Military Courts Fines: Palestinians Imprisoned at Their Own Expense. Institute of Palestine Studies, 11 March. https://www.palestine-studies.org/ar/node/1651045 (accessed 20 May 2021).

44 UNICEF (2020). The Rights of Children Amid COVID-19, May. https://www.unicef.org/sop/reports/rights-children-amid-covid-19.

45 Hagar, S. (2020). Coronavirus 'disaster' at Israeli Factory Prompts Policy Revamp on Palestinian Workers. *Haaretz*, 13 April. https://www.haaretz.com/middle-east-news/ palestinians/.premium-coronavirus-disaster-at-israeli-factory-prompts-revamp-on-palestinian-workers-1.8745545 (accessed 14 April 2020).

46 Medical Aid for Palestinians (MAP) (2017). 'Sometimes patients die': Barriers Facing Palestinian Ambulances Entering East Jerusalem, 24 November. https://www.map.org.uk/news/archive/post/757-athe-aback-to-backa-process-is-hard-and-sometimes-patients-diea-athe-barriers-facing-palestinian-ambulances (accessed 02 July 2020).

47 The World Health Organisation (WHO). COVID-19 Transmission and Protective Measures. https://www.who.int/westernpacific/emergencies/covid-19/information/transmission-protective-measures (accessed 16 May 2021).

48 France 24 (2021). Palestinians Cancel Deal for Near-Expired Covid-19 Vaccine Doses from Israel, 18 June. https://www.france24.com/en

/middle-east/20210618-israel-to-give-palestinians-1-million-soon-to
-expire-covid-19-vaccine-doses-in-exchange-deal (23 June 2021).

49 Al Jazeera (2021). Palestinian Authority Calls off Vaccine Exchange with
    Israel, 18 June. https://www.aljazeera.com/news/2021/6/18/palestinians
    -to-get-1-million-covid-vaccine-doses-in-israel-swap (accessed 26 June
    2021).

50 Shireen Abu Akleh, journalist at Al Jazeera TV. Telephone conversation,
    25 June 2021.

51 Majed, not his real name, media person. Messenger conversation, 24 June
    2021.

52 Ashrawi, Hanan, [@DrHananAshrawi] (2021). If this Isn't Racism &
    Corruption I don't know What is! Israel Uses Palestine as Dumping
    Grounds for Expired Vaccines [. . .], 18 June. https://twitter.com/
    DrHananAshrawi/status/1405959951760113665 (accessed 26 June 2021).

53 Naser-Najjab, N. and Hever, S. (2021). Elite and Popular Contradictions
    in Security Coordination: Overcoming the Binary Distinction of the
    Israeli Coloniser and the Colonised Palestinian. *Critical Studies on
    Security* 9(2): 112–25.

54 The Independent Commission for Human Rights (ICHR). The
    Independent Committee for investigating Vaccine Deal. https://ichr.ps/
    ar/1 (accessed 27 June 2021).

55 Salwa Najjab, MD, is a specialist in obstetrics, gynaecology and
    gynaecological cytology and senior technical advisor at Juzoor
    Foundation Health and Social Development. She is a member of
    the independent fact-finding committee on the Pfizer vaccine and a
    co-founder of several influential grassroots organizations. She is also
    a member of the MENA Health Policy Forum, the Palestinian Health
    Policy Forum and the World Bank Civil Society Consultative Group
    for Health, Nutrition and Population. Personal interview, Exeter, UK,
    04 September 2021.

56 Latin Waves, Grassroot Media. COVID-19 and the Crisis Capitalism
    Creates in Normal Times (Podcast). https://latinwavesmedia.com/
    wordpress/covid19-and-the-crisis-capitalism-creates-in-normal-times/
    (accessed 24 April 2021).

57 Majed, not his real name, media person, Messenger conversation, 24 June
    2021.

58 Fanon, Frantz (1963). *The Wretched of the Earth*. New York: Grove Press; Alfred, Taiaiake (2005). *Wasáse: Indigenous Pathways of Action and Freedom*. Peterborough: Broadview Press. Fanon, F. (2008). *Black Skin, White Masks*. London: Pluto Press.

59 Al-Haq. Al-Haq Position Paper on the Law by Decree Concerning the Amendment of the Law on Charitable Associations and Civil Society Organisations, 10 March 2021. https://www.alhaq.org/advocacy/17959 .html (accessed 17 September 2021).

60 Agamben, Giorgio (2020). The State of Exception Provoked by an Unmotivated Emergency. URL: http://positionswebsite.org/giorgio -agamben-the-state-of-exception-provoked-by-an-unmotivated -emergency/ (accessed 05 February 2021).

61 Agamben, Giorgio (2020). 'Medicine as Religion'. https://itself.blog/2020 /05/02/giorgio-agamben-medicine-as-religion/ (accessed 05 February 2021).

62 Abujidi, Nurhan (2009). The Palestinian States of Exception and Agamben. *Contemporary Arab Affairs* 2(2): 272–91.

63 Hass, Amira (2021). Abbas Tightens His Control over the Palestinian Court System. *Haaretz*, 28 January. https://www.haaretz.com/middle-east -news/palestinians/.premium-sparking-election-fears-abbas-tightens-grip -on-palestinian-court-system-1.9492477 (accessed 30 February 2021).

64 Agamben, Giorgio (2005). *State of Exception*. Translated and edited by Kevin Attell. Chicago: University of Chicago.

65 Foucault, M. (2003). *Society must be Defended: Lectures at the Collège de France, 1975–76*. Translated by David Macey. New York: Picador.

66 Falah, Gh. and Flint, C. (2004). Geopolitical Spaces: The Dialectic of Public and Private Spaces in the Palestine–Israel Conflict. *Arab World Geographer* 7: 11–134.

67 Al-Awsat, Asharq (2021). Shtayyeh: Palestine Received No Financial Aid From US, Arab Countries, 08 April. https://english.aawsat.com/home/ article/2907066/shtayyeh-palestine-received-no-financial-aid-us-arab -countries (accessed 18 July 2021).

68 Clarno, Andy (2017). *Neoliberal Apartheid: Palestine/Israel and South Africa after 1994*. Chicago and London: University of Chicago Press.

69 Tibon, Amir (2018). Trump Administration Released Dozens of Millions of Dollars to Support Palestinian Security Forces. *Haaretz*, 02 August.

https://www.haaretz.com/us-news/.premium-trump-administration
-released-dozens-of-millions-of-dollars-to-pa-1.6340023 (accessed
05 March 2021).

70 Clarno, A. (2017). *Neoliberal Apartheid: Palestine/Israel and South Africa after 1994*. Chicago: University of Chicago Press.

71 Haddad, Toufic (2016). *Palestine Ltd: Neoliberalism and Nationalism in the Occupied Territories*. London: I. B. Taurus.

72 Gramsci, Antonio, Hoare, Quintin and Nowell-Smith, Geoffrey (1971). *Selections from the Prison Notebooks of Antonio Gramsci*. New York: International Publishers.

73 Medical Aid for Palestinians (MAP) (2017). COVID-19 Cases Double again in Palestine: MAP Response Continues, 10 July. https://www.map.org.uk/news/archive/post/1134-covid-19-cases-double-again-in-palestine-map-response-continues (accessed 14 August 2021).

74 Peace to Prosperity Plan (January 2020). Peace-to-Prosperity-0120.pdf (archives.gov) (accessed 07 June 2021).

75 Middle East Eye (2021). Mahmoud Abbas Visits Israeli Defence Minister's Home for Talks, 29 December. https://www.middleeasteye.net/news/israel-palestine-mahmoud-abbas-visits-defence-minister-home-gantz-talks (accessed 06 January 2022).

76 Reuters (2022). Palestinian President, Israeli Defence Minister Meet before Biden Visit, 8 July. https://www.reuters.com/world/middle-east/palestinian-president-israeli-defence-minister-meet-before-biden-visit-2022-07-08/ (accessed 15 August 2022).

77 Israel also previously refused to open Qalandia airport (based between Jerusalem and Ramallah), which operated between 1924 until 1967. It also destroyed the international airport in the Gaza Strip in 2001, just three years after it opened.

78 Abu Toameh, Khaled (2022). Palestinians 'not excited' about Israel's Offer to Use Ramon Airport. *The Jerusalem Post*, 21 July. https://www.jpost.com/arab-israeli-conflict/article-712751 (accessed 09 December 2022).

79 The Office of the European Union Representative (West Bank and Gaza Strip, UNRWA) (2022). The European Union Provides €20 Million to Support the Palestinian COVID-19 Vaccination Campaign, 3 August. https://www.eeas.europa.eu/delegations/palestine-occupied-palestinian

-territory-west-bank-and-gaza-strip/european-union-16_en (accessed 20 August 2022).

80 IMPACT-se (2021). IMPACT-se Review of Georg Eckert Institute (GEI) Report on Palestinian Authority (PA) Textbooks, August.

81 Georg Eckert Institute for International Textbook Research. Report on Palestinian Textbooks. 2021. urn:nbn:de:0220-2021-0020.

82 Starr, Michael (2021). EU Commission Directorate Condemns Antisemitism in Palestinian Textbooks. *Jerusalem Post*, 10 September.

83 The Legal Center for Arab Minority Rights in Israel (ADALA) (2020). Israel Fails to Provide Real-Time Coronavirus Updates in Arabic for Palestinian citizens, 10 March. https://www.adalah.org/en/content/view /9916 (accessed 05 December 2020).

84 Arraf, Suha (2020). Tens of Thousands of Palestinian Citizens in Israel Protest Gun Violence, Organized Crime. +972 Magazine, 04 October. https://www.972mag.com/gun-violence-protest-palestinians-israel /143785/ (accessed 14 January 2021).

85 Derbas, Nahed (2020). The High Level of Crime in the Palestinian Interior under the Auspices of the Occupation Institutions. Al Arabi Al Jadid, 29 December. https://www.alaraby.co.uk/society/h (accessed 02 February 2021).

86 Alzajeera (2021). In Pictures: In Show of Unity, Palestinians Go on Strike, 18 May. https://www.aljazeera.com/gallery/2021/5/18/in-pictures -palestinians-unite-with-a-general-strike (accessed 18 August 2021).

87 Nasasra, M. (2017). *The Naqab Bedouins: A Century of Politics and Resistance.* New York: Columbia University Press.

88 The Jewish National Fund was established by the fifth Zionist Congress in 1901 and tasked with purchasing land in Palestine. It currently owns about 13 per cent of the country's land.

89 Patel, Yumna (2022). What's Happening in the Naqab? Israel Uproots Palestinians to Plant Trees. Mondoweiss, 14 January. https://mondoweiss .net/2022/01/whats-happening-in-the-naqab-israel-uproots-palestinians -to-plant-trees/ (accessed 05 March 2022); in 2004, the Adalah human rights centre for the Arab minority in Israel petitioned the Israeli Supreme Court with the aim of stopping the Fund from discriminating by only allocating land to Jews. The Fund's response helpfully clarified that discrimination is its very raison d'etre. It stated: 'The JNF is not the

trustee of the general public in Israel. Its loyalty is given to the Jewish people in the Diaspora and in the state of Israel. . . . The JNF, in relation to being an owner of land, is not a public body that works for the benefit of all citizens of the state. The loyalty of the JNF is given to the Jewish people and only to them is the JNF obligated. The JNF, as the owner of the JNF land, does not have a duty to practice equality towards all citizens of the state.' Three years later, the Knesset passed the Jewish National Fund Law, which allows the Fund to exclusively allocate land to Jews. This further underlines the Fund's discriminatory character. See Legal Center for Arab Minority Rights in Israel (Adalah) (2007). Land Controlled by Jewish National Fund for Jews Only, 29 July. https://www.adalah.org/en/content/view/6787 (accessed 03 February 2021).

90 Fanon, Frantz (1994). *A Dying Colonialism*. Boston: Grove Atlantic.

91 Hammoudeh, W., Jabr, S., Helbich, M. and Sousa, C. (2020). On Mental Health Amid COVID-19. *Journal of Palestine Studies* 49(4): 77–90.

92 Butler, Judith (2020). Capitalism Has Its Limits. *Verso Books*, 30 March. www.versobooks.com/blogs/4603-capitalism-has-its-limits (accessed 17 May 2020).

93 Hanieh, A. and Ziadah, R. (2022). Pandemic Effects: COVID-19 and the Crisis of Development in the Middle East. *Development and Change* 53(6): 1308–34.

94 The Red Nation. 10 Point Program. https://therednation.org/manifesto/10-point-program/ (accessed 12 April 2019).

95 Agamben, Giorgio (1998). *Homo Sacer: Sovereign Power and Bare Life*. Stanford: Stanford University Press.

96 Mbembe, A. (2003). Necropolitics. *Public Culture* 15(3): 11–40.

97 Mbembe, A. (2003). Necropolitics. *Public Culture* 15(3): 11–40.

98 Weiss, Philip and North, James (2020). Share on Facebook 'We have biblical rights to the land, the Bible is our deed' – Israeli Ambassador Explains Why West Bank belongs to Israel. Mondoweiss, 11 July. https://mondoweiss.net/2020/07/we-have-biblical-rights-to-the-land-the-bible-is-our-deed-israeli-ambassador-explains-why-west-bank-belongs-to-israel/?fbclid=IwAR0qf7WSpQmYTOaFlDSkQj9TjJifyjeL1069oktX_9FNts1kR-ipHX1DyqE (accessed 14 August 2020).

99 France 24 (2021). Netanyahu's Annexation Plan Threatens Palestinian, Israeli Economies Already Struggling after Covid-19, 29 June. https://

www.france24.com/en/20200629-netanyahu-s-annexation-plan
-threatens-palestinian-israeli-economies-already-struggling-after-covid
-19 (accessed 14 July 2021).

100 Peace to Prosperity Plan (January 2020). Peace-to-Prosperity-0120.pdf
(archives.gov) (accessed 14 June 2020).

101 The Biden administration resumed UNRWA funding in April 2021 and
also provided the PA with $15 million to combat Covid-19. See US
Department of State (2021). 'The United States Restores Assistance for
the Palestinians', 7 April. https://www.state.gov/the-united-states-restores
-assistance-for-the-palestinians/ (accessed 02 June 2021).

102 Abu Sneineh, Mustafa (2021). Sheikh Jarrah Explained: The Past and
Present of East Jerusalem Neighbourhood. Middle East Eye, 06 May.
https://www.middleeasteye.net/news/israel-palestine-sheikh-jarrah
-jerusalem-neighbourhood-eviction-explained (accessed 02 June 2021).

103 The Guardian (2021). What has Caused Jerusalem's Worst Violence in
years?, 11 November. https://www.theguardian.com/world/2021/may
/11/what-has-caused-jerusalem-worst-violence-in-years-israel-palestine
(accessed 02 December 2021).

104 Naser-Najjab, Nadia (2021). My Teenage Nephew was Beaten by Israeli
Forces – Sadly, this is not an Isolated Case. Middle East Eye, 7 June.
https://www.middleeasteye.net/opinion/israel-palestine-east-jerusalem
-teenage-beaten-not-unusual (accessed 02 October 2021).

105 Naser-Najjab, Nadia (2022). A Message from Palestinians to Abbas:
Concessions to Israel only Elicit more Demands, 6 January. https://www
.middleeasteye.net/opinion/israel-palestine-burqa-concessions-elicit
-more-demands (accessed 21 April 2022).

106 Wolfe, Patrick (1999). *Settler Colonialism and the Transformation of
Anthropology: The Politics and Poetics of and Ethnographic Event.* London:
Cassell. Wolfe, Patrick (2006). Settler Colonialism and the Elimination of
the Native. *Journal of Genocide Research* 8(4): 388–9. Veracini, Lorenzo
(2010). *Settler Colonialism: A Theoretical Overview.* Basingstoke: Palgrave
Macmillan. Veracini, Lorenzo (2011). Introducing. *Settler Colonial
Studies* 1(1): 1–12. Mamdani, Mahmood (2015). Settler Colonialism:
Then and Now. *Critical Inquiry* 41(3): 596–614.

107 Lustick, Ian (1980). *Arabs in the Jewish State: Israel's Control of a National
Minority.* Austin: Texas University Press. Ghanem, As'ad and Mustafa,

Muhannad (2008). *Palestinians in Israel*. Madar: Ramallah. Pappe, Ilan (2020). *The Biggest Prison on Earth: A History of the Occupied Territories*. London: Oneworld Publications.

108　Mbembe, A. (2003). Necropolitics. *Public Culture* 15(3): 11–40.

109　Smith, Linda Tuhiwai (2012). *Decolonizing Methodologies*. London: Zed Books. Abu-Saad, I. (2008). Where Inquiry Ends: The Peer Review Process and Indigenous Standpoints. *American Behavioral Scientist* 51: 1902–18.

110　Onyango, Joel and Ndege, Nora (2021). How Do We 'Decolonise' Research Methodologies? STEPS Centre, 10 March. https://steps-centre .org/blog/how-do-we-decolonise-research-methodologies/ (accessed 02 July 2021).

111　The Forum, which was established on 10 April 2018, brings together Palestinian intellectuals, academics, artists and activists from the oPt, Israel and other countries. It organizes workshops and seminars and invites speakers to exchange ideas and views on rebuilding Palestinian institutions and developing future solutions to various challenges, including the Sheikh Jarrah stand-off. I became a member of its coordinating and intellectual committees at the end of 2020.

112　Tamari, S. (1995). Tourists with Agendas. *Middle East Report* 196: 25.

113　Al-Hardan, A. (2014). Decolonizing Research on Palestinians: Towards Critical Epistemologies and Research Practices. *Qualitative Inquiry* 20(1): 66.

114　Al-mughrabi, Nidal and Heller, Jeffrey (2021). Gaza Tower Block Collapses after Israeli Air Strike, Witnesses Say. *Reuters*, 11 May. https:// www.reuters.com/world/middle-east/palestinian-rocket-fire-israeli-air -strikes-gaza-2021-05-11/ (accessed 02 August 2021).

115　Al-Hardan, A. (2014). Decolonizing Research on Palestinians: Towards Critical Epistemologies and Research Practices. *Qualitative Inquiry* 20(1): 67.

116　Smith, Linda Tuhiwai (2012) *Decolonizing Methodologies*. Zed Books.

117　Peace to Prosperity Plan (January 2020). Peace-to-Prosperity-0120.pdf (archives.gov) (accessed 14 June 2020).

118　Khalidi refers to the Accords as a collection of 'phraseological tricks', whose true intent was 'concealed by a veil of deceitful, Orwellian verbiage'. See Khalidi, Rashid (2012). *Brokers of Deceit – How the US Has Undermined Peace in the Middle East*. Boston: Beacon Press, 28.

119 Weiss, Philip (2020). 'Whether they Accept It or not, It's Going to Happen' – Netanyahu Lays Out Palestinian Submission to Trump Plan. Mondoweiss. 18 February. https://mondoweiss.net/2020/02/ whether-they-accept-it-or-not-its-going-to-happen-netanyahu-lays-out -palestinian-submission-to-trump-plan/?fbclid=IwAR3bE5aGgE6Jl5uJG ZO5adxqk1TdjQ-fhwo6kxqGyhi7FUM6CaTIBUgDNuQ.

120 Naser-Najjab, N. (2020). Palestinian Leadership and the Contemporary Significance of the First Intifada. *Race & Class* 62(2): 61–79.

121 Peace to Prosperity Plan (January 2020). Peace-to-Prosperity-0120.pdf (archives.gov) (accessed 14 June 2020).

122 Naser-Najjab, Nadia (2019). The Oslo People-to-People Program and the Limits of Hegemony. *Middle East Critique* 28(4): 425–43.

123 B'Tselem (2018). The Israeli Information Center for Human Rights in the Occupied Territories Three Israeli Supreme Court Justices Greenlight State to Commit War Crime, 27 May. https://www.btselem.org/ communities_facing_expulsion/20180527_supreme_court_greenlights _war_crime_in_khan_al_ahmar (accessed 15 August 2022).

124 Sabbagh-Khoury, A. (2021). Tracing Settler Colonialism: A Genealogy of a Paradigm in the Sociology of Knowledge Production in Israel. *Politics & Society* 50(1): 1–40.

Chapter 1

1 Fanon, Frantz (1994). *A Dying Colonialism*. Boston: Grove Atlantic.

2 Pappé, Ilan (2017). *Ten Myths About Israel*. London: Verso Books. Weizman, Eyal (2007). *Hollow Land: Israel's Architecture of Occupation*. London: Verso Books.

3 Trouillot, Michel-Rolph (2015). *Silencing the Past: Power and the Production of History*, 2nd revised edn. Boston: Beacon Press.

4 Sayegh, Fayez (1965). *Zionist Colonialism in Palestine, 1965*. Beirut: Research Center, Palestine Liberation Organization.

5 Amensty International (2022). Israel's Apartheid against Palestinians: A Cruel System of Domination and a Crime against Humanity, 1 February. https://www.amnesty.org/en/latest/news/2022/02/israels-apartheid

-against-palestinians-a-cruel-system-of-domination-and-a-crime-against
-humanity/ (accessed 02 April 2021).

6 Wolfe, P. (2006). Settler-Colonialism and the Elimination of the Native. *Journal of Genocide Research* 8(4): 387–409.

7 Any reflection on this international dimension should also consider the role and contribution of regional actors. For example, refer to the historical example of the Arab League's establishment of an Arab higher executive in 1946. It selected members on the basis of class and family, which ultimately resulted in a relatively moderate strategy that included sending delegates to Britain, so they would contribute to strike actions. By implication, the executive did not develop a counter-colonial strategy or establish an organized popular base within historical Palestine. See Hilal, Jamil (2002). *The Formation of the Palestinian Elite: From the Palestinian National Movement to the Rise of the Palestinian Authority* (in Arabic), the Palestinian Institute for the Study of Democracy (Muwatin).

8 Also see Kaplan (2018).

9 Said, Edward (2001). Introduction. In Said, E. W. and Hitchens, C. (eds), *Blaming the Victims: Spurious Scholarship and the Palestinian Question.* New York: Verso. Kaplan, A. (2018). *Our American Israel: The Story of an Entangled Alliance.* Cambridge, MA: Harvard University Press.

10 Sayegh, Fayez (1965). *Zionist Colonialism in Palestine, 1965.* Beirut: Research Center, Palestine Liberation Organization.

11 Rishmawi, Mona (1986). Planning in Whose Interest? Land Use Planning as a Strategy for Judaization. Al-Haq Organization.

12 B'Tselem – The Israeli Information Center for Human Rights in the Occupied Territories. Israel Destroys Palestinian Farmland in Gaza again, Allegedly for Security, 12 November 2020. https://www.btselem .org/video/20201112_israel_destroys_palestinian_farmland_in_gaza _again#full (accessed 21 February 2021).

13 Weizman, Eyal (2007). *Hollow Land: Israel's Architecture of Occupation.* London: Verso Books. Halper, J. (2015). *War Against the People: Israel, the Palestinians and Global Pacification.* London: Pluto Press.

14 Badarin, Emile (2015). Settler-Colonialist Management of Entrances to the Native Urban Space in Palestine. *Settler Colonial Studies* 5(3): 226–35.

15 Badarin, Emile (2015). Settler-Colonialist Management of Entrances to the Native Urban Space in Palestine. *Settler Colonial Studies* 5(3): 226–35.

Weizman, Eyal (2007). *Hollow Land: Israel's Architecture of Occupation*. London: Verso Books. Halper, J. (2015). *War Against the People: Israel, the Palestinians and Global Pacification*. London: Pluto Press.

16 Roy, Sara (2004). The Palestinian-Israeli Conflict and Palestinian Socioeconomic Decline: A Place Denied. *International Journal of Politics, Culture, and Society* 17, no. 3 (Spring): 365–403.

17 Hilal, Jamil (2015). Rethinking Palestine: Settler-Colonialism, Neoliberalism and Individualism in the West Bank and Gaza Strip. *Contemporary Arab Affairs*. DOI: 10.1080/17550912.2015.1052226.

18 Farsakh, Leila (2008). Independence, Cantons or Bantustans: Whither the Palestinian State? *Middle East Journal* 59, no. 2 (Spring): 238.

19 Tufajki, Khalil (2000). Settlements: A Geographic and Demographic Barrier to Peace. *Palestine-Israel Journal, of Political, Economics and Culture* 7(3 and 4): 52–8.

20 Weizman, Eyal (2007). *Hollow Land: Israel's Architecture of Occupation*. London: Verso Books. Halper, J. (2015). *War Against the People: Israel, the Palestinians and Global Pacification*. London: Pluto Press.

21 Wolfe, P. (2006). 'Settler-Colonialism and the Elimination of the Native'. *Journal of Genocide Research* 8(4): 388.

22 Peace Now: 123% Increase in Settlement Construction in 2013, 3 March 2014. https://972mag.com/nstt_feeditem/peace-now-123-increase-in -settlement-construction-in-2013/.

23 The New Declared Settlement Policy (2017). Not a Restraint at All, Peace Now, 31 March. http://peacenow.org.il/en/new-declared-settlement -policy-not-restraint (accessed 19 June 2021).

24 Weizman, Eyal (2007). *Hollow Land: Israel's Architecture of Occupation*. London: Verso.

25 Hilal, Jamil (2015). Rethinking Palestine: Settler-Colonialism, Neoliberalism and Individualism in the West Bank and Gaza Strip. *Contemporary Arab Affairs*. doi: 10.1080/17550912.2015.1052226.

26 Hilal, Jamil (2015). Rethinking Palestine: Settler-Colonialism, Neoliberalism and Individualism in the West Bank and Gaza Strip. *Contemporary Arab Affairs*. doi: 10.1080/17550912.2015.1052226.

27 United Nations (2006). *Report of the Special Rapporteur of the Commission on Human Rights, John Dugard, on the Situation of Human Rights in the Palestinian Territories Occupied by Israel Since 1967*, United

Nations Commission on Human Rights, UN Doc. E/CN.4/2006/29, 17 January.

28 Farsakh, Leila (2008). Independence, Cantons or Bantustans: Whither the Palestinian State? *Middle East Journal* 59, no. 2 (Spring): 238.

29 Roy, S. (1995). *The Gaza Strip: The Political Economy of De-Development.* Washington, DC: Institute for Palestinian Studies.

30 Alfred, Taiaiake (1999). *Peace, Power, Righteousness: An Indigenous Manifesto.* New York: Oxford University Press.

31 Veracini, Lorenzo (2010). *Settler Colonialism: A Theoretical Overview.* Basingstoke: Palgrave Macmillan.

32 Veracini, Lorenzo (2011). Introducing. *Settler Colonial Studies* 1(1): 1–12.

33 Veracini, Lorenzo (2010). *Settler Colonialism: A Theoretical Overview.* Basingstoke: Palgrave Macmillan.

34 Jerusalem Media & Communications Centre (JMCC) (1993). Israeli Military Orders in the Occupied Palestinian West Bank (1967-1992). Jerusalem, JMCC.

35 Rishmawi, Mona (1986). Planning in Whose Interest? Land Use Planning as a Strategy for Judaization. Al-Haq Organization. Tamari, Salim (1988). What the Uprising Means. Middle East Report, No. 152. *The Uprising,* 24–30.

36 Hilal, Jamil (2015). Rethinking Palestine: Settler-Colonialism, Neoliberalism and Individualism in the West Bank and Gaza Strip. *Contemporary Arab Affairs.* DOI: 10.1080/17550912.2015.1052226. Roy, Sara (2004). The Palestinian-Israeli Conflict and Palestinian Socioeconomic Decline: A Place Denied. *International Journal of Politics, Culture, and Society* 17(3): 365–403.

37 Memmi, A. (1974). *The Colonizer and the Colonized.* London: Souvenir Press.

38 Badarin, E. (2016). *Palestinian Political Discourse, between Exile and Occupation.* London: Routledge, 159.

39 Quray', Aḥmad (2005). *al-Riwāyah al-Filasṭīnīyah al-kāmilah lil-mufāwaḍāt: min Ūslū ilá Kharīṭat al-ṭarīq.* Vol. 1. Bayrūt: Mu'assasat al-Dirāsāt al-Filasṭīnīyah.

40 Quray', Aḥmad (2005). *al-Riwāyah al-Filasṭīnīyah al-kāmilah lil-mufāwaḍāt: min Ūslū ilá Kharīṭat al-ṭarīq.* Vol. 1. Bayrūt: Mu'assasat al-Dirāsāt al-Filasṭīnīyah.

41 Quray', Aḥmad (2005). *al-Riwāyah al-Filasṭīnīyah al-kāmilah lil-mufāwaḍāt: min Ūslū ilá Kharīṭat al-ṭarīq.* Vol. 1. Bayrūt: Mu'assasat al-Dirāsāt al-Filasṭīnīyah, 101.

42 In April 2014, Israel also objected to Palestinian attempts to form a unity government.

43 Savir, Uri (1998). *The Process: 1,100 days that Changed the Middle East.* New York: Random House, 102.

44 Quray', Aḥmad (2005). *al-Riwāyah al-Filasṭīnīyah al-kāmilah lil-mufāwaḍāt: min Ūslū ilá Kharīṭat al-ṭarīq.* Vol. 1. Bayrūt: Mu'assasat al-Dirāsāt al-Filasṭīnīyah, 305.

45 Ahren, Rapheal (2014). Netanyahu: Abbas must choose between Israel and Hamas. *The Times of Israel*, 23 April. https://www.timesofisrael.com /netanyahu-abbas-must-choose-between-israel-and-hamas/ (accessed 07 June 2021). See also, PLO and Israeli Letters of Mutual Recognition, Tunis and Jerusalem, 9 September 1993. *JPS* 23, no. 1 (Autumn 1993): 114–15, 115.

46 Bishara, Marwan (2001). *Palestine/Israel: Peace or Apartheid: Occupation, Terrorism and the Future.* London: Zed Books, 56.

47 Hammami, Rema and Hilal, Jamil (2001). An Uprising at a Crossroads. *Middle East Report*, No. 219 (Summer): 2-7+41. For impact of second Intifada on Palestinian lives, see Roy, Sara (2004). The Palestinian-Israeli Conflict and Palestinian Socioeconomic Decline: A Place Denied. *International Journal of Politics, Culture and Society* 17(3): 365–403, and World Bank (2007). *Movement and Access Restrictions in the West Bank and Gaza Strip: Uncertainty and Insufficiency in the Palestine Economy.* Washington D.C. World Bank. http://siteresources .worldbank.org/INTWESTBANKGAZA/Resources/WestBankrestric tions9Mayfinal.pdf (accessed 09 June 2020).

48 Levy, Gideon. Israel Endangers Jewish Lives. *Ha'aretz*, 17 August 2003.

49 Roy, S. (2011). *Hamas and Civil Society in Gaza: Engaging the Islamist Social Sector.* Princeton and Oxford: Princeton University Press.

50 Hilal, Jamil (2015). Rethinking Palestine: Settler-Colonialism, Neoliberalism and Individualism in the West Bank and Gaza Strip. *Contemporary Arab Affairs.* DOI: 10.1080/17550912.2015.1052226.

51 Fanon, Frantz (1963). *The Wretched of the Earth.* New York: Grove Press.

52 Hilal, Jamil (2010). *The Pauperization of Women, Men and Children in the West Bank and Gaza Strip.* Birzeit: Institute for Women's Studies, Birzeit University.

53 Fanon, Frantz (1963). *The Wretched of the Earth.* New York: Grove Press.

54 Badarin, Emile (2015). Settler-Colonialist Management of Entrances to the Native Urban Space in Palestine. *Settler Colonial Studies* 5(3): 226–35.

55 Pappé, Ilan (2013). Revisiting 1967: The False Paradigm of Peace, Partition and Parity. *Settler Colonial Studies* 3(3–4): 341–51.

56 Tartir, Alaa (2015). The Evolution and Reform of Palestinian Security Forces 1993–2013. *Stability: International Journal of Security and Development* 4(1): 1–20.

57 Clarno, Andy (2017). *Neoliberal Apartheid: Palestine/Israel and South Africa after 1994.* Chicago and London: University of Chicago Press.

58 Fast, Larissa (2006). Aid in the Pressure Cooker Humanitarian Action in the Occupied Palestinian Territory. *Humanitarian Agenda*, Case Study no. 7. Boston: Feinstein International Center.

59 Abdalla, Hisham (2017). Palestinians Protest over PA-Israel Security Ties. *Al-Jazeera*, 14 March.

60 Swisher, Clayton E. (2011). *The Palestine Papers: The End of the Road.* London: Hesperus Press.

61 Israel also (most recently on 18 August 2022) raided the premises of civil society organizations and destroyed equipment and confiscated materials. They were closed them and signs (reading 'unlawful') and orders ('security in the region, & to combat the infrastructure of terrorism') on their doors. This was clearly intended to break Palestinian resistance.
    See Addameer – الضمير [@Addameer]. (18 August 2022). BREAKING: this morning Israeli occupation forces raided the offices of Addameer, as well as @alhaq_org @bisanresearch @UAWC1986 & @of committees [Tweet]. Twitter. https://twitter.com/Addameer/status/1560126708916830210 (accessed 20 August 2022). Our doors were broken down, material confiscated, and a military order left behind. #StandWithThe6.

62 The Guardian, Palestinian Unity Government of Fatah and Hamas Sworn in 2 June 2014. https://www.theguardian.com/world/2014/jun/02/palestinian-unity-government-sworn-in-fatah-Hamas (accessed 14 January 2020).

63 Coulthard, Glen S. (2014). *Red Skin, White Masks: Rejecting the Colonial Politics of Recognition.* Minneapolis: University of Minnesota Press.

64 Coulthard, Glen S. (2014). *Red Skin, White Masks: Rejecting the Colonial Politics of Recognition*. Minneapolis: University of Minnesota Press.

65 Fanon, F. (1967 [1964]). *Toward the African Revolution*. Translated by Haakon Chevalier. New York: Grove Press.

66 Mbembe, A. (2003). Necropolitics. *Public Culture* 15(3): 11–40.

67 Dunbar-Ortiz, R. and Gilio-Whitaker, D. (2016). *'All the Real Indians Died Off': And 20 Other Myths about Native Americans*. Beacon Press.

68 Fanon, Frantz (1963). *The Wretched of the Earth*. New York: Grove Press.

69 Veracini, Lorenzo (2010). *Settler Colonialism: A Theoretical Overview*. Basingstoke: Palgrave Macmillan. Makdisi, S. (2010). *Palestine Inside Out: An Everyday Occupation*. New York: Norton.

70 Pappé, Ilan (2017). *Ten Myths About Israel*. London and New York: Verso Books.

71 Memmi, Albert (1974). *The Colonizer and the Colonized*. London: Souvenir Press.

72 Hilal, Jamil (2015). Rethinking Palestine: Settler-Colonialism, Neoliberalism and Individualism in the West Bank and Gaza Strip. *Contemporary Arab Affairs*. doi: 10.1080/17550912.2015.1052226.

73 Rouhana, Nadim and Sabbagh-Khoury, Areej (2015). Settler-Colonial Citizenship: Conceptualizing the Relationship between Israel and Its Palestinian Citizens. *Settler Colonial Studies* 5(3): 41. Nasasra, Mansour et al. (2015). The Naqab Bedouin and Colonialism. *New Perspectives*, 1–32.

74 Abed Elrazik, Adnan, Amin, Riyad and Davis, Uri (Spring 1978). Problems of Palestinians in Israel, Land, Work, Education. *Journal of Palestine Studies* 7(3): 31–54.

75 Adalah (2020). The Legal Center for Arab Minority Rights. Israel's Jewish Nation-State Law, 20 December. https://www.adalah.org/en/content/view/9569 (accessed 23 February 2021).

76 Jabareen, Hassan and Bishara, Suhad (2019). The Jewish Nation-State Law. *Journal of Palestine Studies* 48(2): 43–57.

77 The Legal Center for Arab Minority Rights in Israel (ADALA) (2014). Israeli Supreme Court upholds 'Admissions Committees Law' that Allows Israeli Jewish Communities to Exclude Palestinian Arab Citizens, 17 September. https://www.adalah.org/en/content/view/8327 (accessed 05 December 2020).

78 Rouhana, Nadim and Sabbagh-Khoury, Areej (2015). Settler-Colonial
    Citizenship: Conceptualizing the Relationship between Israel and Its
    Palestinian Citizens. *Settler Colonial Studies* 5(3): 41 Nasasra, Mansour
    et al. (2015). The Naqab Bedouin and Colonialism. *New Perspectives*
    1–32. Nasasra, M. (2017). *The Naqab Bedouins: A Century of Politics and
    Resistance.* Columbia University Press.

79 Badarin, Emile (2015). Settler-Colonialist Management of Entrances to
    the Native Urban Space in Palestine. *Settler Colonial Studies* 5(3): 226–35.

80 Foucault, M. (2003a). *Society must be Defended: Lectures at the Collège de
    France, 1975–76.* Picador.

81 Agamben, Giorgio (1998). *Homo Sacer: Sovereign Power and Bare Life.*
    Stanford: Stanford University Press.

82 Agamben, Giorgio (2020). Clarifications, 17 March 2020. https://medium
    .com/@ddean3000/clarifications-giorgio-agamben-3f97dc7ed67c.

83 Tawil-Souri, H. (2011). Colored Identity: The Politics and Materiality of
    ID Cards in Palestine/Israel. *Social Text* 29(2): 67–97.

84 Foucault, M. (2003a). *Society must be Defended: Lectures at the Collège de
    France, 1975–76.* Picador.

85 Foucault, Michel (2003b). *Abnormal. Lectures at the Collége de France
    1974-1975.* Translated by Graham Burchell. London and New York:
    Verso Books.

86 Foucault, Michel (1990). *The History of Sexuality, Vol. 1, An Introduction.*
    Translated by Robert Hurley. London: Penguin Books.

87 Foucault, M. (1978). *The History of Sexuality.* New York: Vintage.

88 Foucault, M. (1991). *Discipline and Punish: The Birth of a Prison.*
    London: Penguin.

89 Morgensen, Scott Lauria (2013). The Biopolitics of Settler Colonialism:
    Right Here, Right Now. *Settler Colonial Studies* 1(1): 52–76.

90 Daher-Nashif, S. (2021). Colonial Management of Death: To be or not to
    be Dead in Palestine. *Current Sociology* 69(7): 945–62.

91 Foucault, Michel (1990). *History of Sexuality Vol. 1, An Introduction.* New
    York: Vintage.

92 Foucault, M. (1978). *The History of Sexuality.* New York: Vintage.

93 Silverstein, Richard (2020). Israel Is Militarizing and Monetizing the
    COVID-19 Pandemic. *Jacobin*, 16 April. https://jacobinmag.com/2020/4/
    israel-military-surveillance-coronavirus-covid-netanyahu.

94 Shalhoub-Kevorkian, N. (2015). *Security Theology, Surveillance and the Politics of Fear*. Cambridge Studies in Law and Society, Cambridge: Cambridge University Press.

95 Shalhoub-Kevorkian, N. (2015). *Security Theology, Surveillance and the Politics of Fear*. Cambridge Studies in Law and Society, Cambridge: Cambridge University Press.

96 Ghanim, H. (2008). Thanatopolitics: The Case of the Colonial Occupation in Palestine. In R. Lentin (ed.), *Thinking Palestine*, 65–81. London: Zed Books.

97 B'Tselem (2021). Since Pandemic, has Israel Allowed almost no Palestinians Out of Gaza for Medical Treatment, 03 May. https://www .btselem.org/gaza_strip/20210503_gaza_patients_denied_treatment _since_covid_19_outbreak (accessed 03 November 2021).

98 Chamberlin, Paul (2011). The Struggle against Oppression Everywhere: The Global Politics of Palestinian Liberation. *Middle Eastern Studies* 47(1): 25–41.

99 Davis, Angela Y. (2016). *Freedom Is a Constant Struggle: Ferguson, Palestine, and the Foundations of a Movement*. Chicago: Haymarket Books.

100 Waziyatawin (2012). Malice Enough in their Hearts and Courage Enough in Ours: Reflections on US Indigenous and Palestinian Experiences under Occupation. *Settler Colonial Studies* 2(1): 172–89.

101 Salamanca, O. J., Qato, M., Rabie, K. and Samour, S. (2012). Past is Present: Settler Colonialism in Palestine. *Settler Colonial Studies* 2(1): 1–8.

102 Dunbar-Ortiz, Roxanne (2014). *An Indigenous Peoples' History of the United States*. Boston: Beacon Press.

103 Coulthard, Glen S. (2014). *Red Skin, White Masks: Rejecting the Colonial Politics of Recognition*. Minneapolis: University of Minnesota Press.

104 Coulthard, Glen S. (2014). *Red Skin, White Masks: Rejecting the Colonial Politics of Recognition* Minneapolis: University of Minnesota Press.

105 Alfred, Taiaiake (2005). *Wasáse: Indigenous Pathways of Action and Freedom*. University of Toronto Press.

106 Simpson, Leanne (2011). *Dancing on Our Turtle's Back: Stories of Nishnaabeg Re-Creation, Resurgence and a New Emergence*. Winnipeg: Arbeiter Ring Press.

107 Idle No More. Vision. https://idlenomore.ca/about-the-movement/ (accessed 22 July 2021).

108　Native News Online (2020). In Landmark Decision, Supreme Court Rules that Nearly Half of Oklahoma is Indian Land, 09 July. https:// nativenewsonline.net/currents/in-landmark-decision-supreme -court-rules-that-nearly-half-of-oklahoma-is-indian-land (accessed 23 February 2021).

109　Dunbar-Ortiz, Roxanne (2014). *An Indigenous Peoples' History of the United States*. Boston: Beacon Press.

110　Nasrallah, Elias (2016). *Testimonies on the First Century of Palestine*. Beirut: Dar Al-Farabi.

111　Fanon, Frantz (1963) *The Wretched of the Earth*. New York: Grove Press.

112　Tuck, Eve and Yang, K. Yayne (2012). Decolonization is not a Metaphor. *Decolonization: Indigeneity, Education & Society*1(1): 1–40.

113　Qumsiyeh, Mazin B. (2016). A Critical and Historical Assessment of Boycott, Divestment, and Sanctions (BDS) in Palestine. In Ozerdem, Alpaslan, Thiessen, Chuck and Qassoum, Mufid (eds), *Conflict Transformation and the Palestinians*. Florence: Taylor and Francis, chapter 5, 89–113.

114　Hilal, Jamil (2015). Rethinking Palestine: Settler-Colonialism, Neoliberalism and Individualism in the West Bank and Gaza Strip. *Contemporary Arab Affairs*. doi: 10.1080/17550912.2015.1052226.

115　Union of Agricultural Work Committees (2020). UAWC distributing Food Baskets and Hygiene Kits for 400 Affected Families from Covid-19 in GAZA, 22 October.

116　Nasr Abdul Karim (2020). āltdāʿyāt ālāqtṣādyᵊ lāntšar wbāʾ kwrwnā fy flsṭynᶜ wāltdḫlāt ālāqtṣādyᵊ ālmtāḥᵊ fy ftrᵊ ālwbāʾ (The Economic Repercussions of the Coronavirus Pandemic in Palestine, and the Available Economic Interventions during the Pandemic Period). *Masarat - The Palestinian Center for Policy Research & Strategic Studies*, 10 October. https://www.masarat.ps/article/ (accessed 06 January 2022).

117　Union of Agricultural Work Committees (2020). The Union of Agricultural Work Committees Finishes the Distribution of 500 Hygiene Kits and Awareness Brochures in 10 Communities in the West Bank, as Part of the Third Phase of Its Campaign 'UnitedAgainstCOVID-19', 04 May. https://uawc-pal.org/news.php?n=3590&lang=2 (accessed 23 August 2022).

118 La Via Campesina – A Movement of Movements and the Global Voice of Peasants1 Who Feed the World. https://viacampesina.org/en/international-peasants-voice/ (accessed 23 August 2022).

119 In the first year of the *Intifada,* I volunteered with Medical Relief Committee in a campaign to test blood types. We issued a card with people's blood type, which also enabled them to donate blood to the injured. I also undertook a first aid training in response to a UNLU call 'for an expansion of the work of the health committees, and for an increase in the organization of first aid courses and preventive medicine and health education'.

120 Giacaman, Rita (2018, February 1). Reframing Public Health in Wartime: From the Biomedical Model to the 'Wounds Inside'. *Journal of Palestine Studies* 47(2): 9–27.

121 UN News (2020). Envoy Welcomes Restart of Israeli-Palestinian Coordination Amid COVID-19 Rise, 18 November. https://news.un.org/en/story/2020/11/1077942 (accessed 23 April 2021).

122 Naser-Najjab, Nadia (2020). *Dialogue in Palestine: The People-to-People Diplomacy Programme and the Israeli-Palestinian Conflict.* Bloomsbury Publishing.

123 Levy, Gideon and Levak, Alex (2021). It's Not the First Time a Palestinian Dies This Way During a Nighttime Israeli Army Raid. *Haaretz*, 11 March. https://www.haaretz.com/israel-news/.premium .MAGAZINE-it-s-not-the-first-time-a-palestinian-dies-this-way -during-a-nighttime-idf-raid-1.9613030?fbclid=IwAR3sSNny6ZIi0 CFVdTd7xriQB0XCMXRAmma_G-7HPDkwpm3PSduiXhXi7vA (accessed 20 October 2021).

124 Health Sector Signatories, Occupied Palestine | Palestinian Committee for the Academic and Cultural Boycott of Israel (2005). An Open Letter to the Palestinian and International Community Regarding Palestinian-Israeli Cooperation in Health. http://www.monabaker.com/pMachine/more.php?id=2903_0_1_84_M5 (accessed 20 February 2020).

125 Health Sector Signatories, Occupied Palestine | Palestinian Committee for the Academic and Cultural Boycott of Israel (2005). An Open Letter to the Palestinian and International Community Regarding Palestinian-Israeli Cooperation in Health. http://www.monabaker.com/pMachine/more.php?id=2903_0_1_84_M5 (accessed 20 February 2020).

126 Hammami, Rema (1995). NGOs: The Professionalization of Politics. *Race & Class* 37(2): 51–63.

127 Muaddi, Qassam (2021). Palestinian Authority's Push to Regulate NGOs Raises Fear of Power Grab. Middle East Eye 03 March. https://www.middleeasteye.net/news/abbas-new-law-will-turn-palestinian-nonprofits-government-agencies-according-palestinian-ngos?fbclid=IwAR3J0Q16cT0PY-bL-jJNK2myARAsQMPGRvcMp45f_CXo-peYLjl7RyHoD0w (accessed 23 November 2021).

128 Roy, S. (1999). De-development Revisited: Palestinian Economy and Society since Oslo. *Journal of Palestine Studies* 28(3): 64–82.

129 Khatib, R., Mataria, A., Donaldson, C., Bossert, T., Hunter, D. J., Alsayed, F. and Moatti, J. P. (2009, April 4). The Health-Care System: An Assessment and Reform Agenda. *Lancet* 373(9670): 1207–17. DOI: 10.1016/S0140-6736(09)60111-2. Epub 2009 March 4. PMID: 19268349.

130 Pappe, Ilan (2017). *The Biggest Prison on Earth: A History of the Occupied Territories.* London: Oneworld Publications. Hanieh, Adam. Palestine in the Middle East: Opposing Neoliberalism and US Power. *MRzine*, 19 July 2008. http://www.monthlyreview.org/mrzine.

131 NGO Monitor (2020). In a First, EU to Investigate if Funding Went to Terror Linked NGOs, 20 May. https://www.ngo-monitor.org/eu-to-investigate-funding-terror-linked-ngos/ (accessed 23 November 2020).

132 Dana, Tareq (2020). Criminalizing Palestinian Resistance: The EU's Additional Condition on Aid to Palestine. *Al Shabaka*, 02 February. https://al-shabaka.org/commentaries/criminalizing-palestinian-resistance-the-eu-new-conditions-on-aid-to-palestine/ (16 May 2020).

133 Harkov, Lahav (2021). EU Moves to Stop Funding Palestinian Terrorists, Inciting Textbooks. *The Jerusalem Post*, 18 April. https://www.jpost.com/arab-israeli-conflict/eu-moves-to-stop-funding-palestinian-terrorists-inciting-textbooks-666595 (accessed 09 June 2021).

134 Pappé, Ilan (2006). *The Ethnic Cleansing of Palestine.* Oxford: Oneworld.

135 Sitta also observes that in 1955 Ben Gurion sought to develop 'a cheap non-conventional capability' that could be used against the Egyptians during hostilities that followed a year later. See Abu Sitta, Salman (2003). Traces of Poison – Israel's Dark History Revealed. *Ahram Weekly*, 27 February—5 March. https://www.plands.org/en/articles-speeches/articles/2003/traces-of-poison%E2%80%93israels-dark-history-revealed

(accessed 18 October 2022). In the contemporary context, Israel's use of unconventional weapons includes the use of white phosphorous, as during 2009 attacks on the Strip. See Human Rights Watch. Rain of Fire: Israel's Unlawful Use of White Phosphorus in Gaza, 25 March 2009. https://www.hrw.org/report/2009/03/25/rain-fire/israels-unlawful-use-white-phosphorus-gaza (accessed 19 October 2022).

136 Morris, B. and Kedar, B. Z. (2022). 'Cast thy bread': Israeli Biological Warfare during the 1948 War. *Middle Eastern Studies*, 1–25. doi: 10.1080/00263206.2022.2122448

137 Rigby, Andrew (1991). *Living the Intifada*. London: Zed Books.

138 Boxerman, Aaron (2021). With Distrust Rampant, East Jerusalem Palestinians shirk COVID Vaccine. *The Times of Israel*, 06 January. https://www.timesofisrael.com/with-distrust-rampant-east-jerusalem-palestinians-shirk-covid-vaccine/ (accessed 23 June 2021).

139 Middle East Monitor (MEMO) (2020). Palestinian Medical Group Threatens to Step Up Protests against Government, 27 February. https://www.middleeastmonitor.com/20200227-palestinian-medical-group-threatens-to-step-up-protests-against-government/ (accessed 20 December 2020).

140 Middle East Monitor (MEMO) (2020). US Provides $500m to Israel under National Covid Relief Bill, 22 December. https://www.middleeastmonitor.com/20201222-us-provides-500m-to-israel-under-national-covid-relief-bill/?fbclid=IwAR37VmJhSuP7HAY4VJ-uisb_9uoMXh_rEnFxLOHxFd8tbCBMu8y29pscLdM (accessed 23 December 2020).

141 The Jerusalem Post. 100 Ventilators Arrive to Israel from the U.S, 15 April 2020. https://www.jpost.com/breaking-news/100-ventilators-arrive-to-israel-from-the-us-624718 (accessed 05 February 2021). Abunimah, Ali (2020). Did the U.S. Just Supply a Million Face Masks to the Israeli Army? *Electronic Intifada*, 8 April. https://electronicintifada.net/blogs/ali-abunimah/did-us-just-supply-million-face-masks-israeli-army (accessed 05 February 2021).

142 Rasgon, Adam and Kingsley, Patrick (2021). As Palestinians Clamor for Vaccine, Their Leaders Divert Doses to Favored Few. *The New York Times*, 03 March. https://www.nytimes.com/2021/03/03/world/middleeast/Palestinians-Israel-vaccine-favoritism.html (accessed 14 July 2021).

143 The Coalition for Accountability and Integrity – AMAN, 27 February 2021. https://www.aman-palestine.org/activities/14812.html (accessed 27 March 2021).

144 Dignified we Stand. http://waqfetizz.ps/en (03 April 2021).

145 Dunbar-Ortiz, Ronanne (2014). *An Indigenous Peoples' History of the United States*. Boston: Beacon Press.

146 Muzembo, B. A., Ntontolo, N. P., Ngatu, N. R., Khatiwada, J., Ngombe, K. L., Numbi, O. L., Nzaji, K. M., Maotela, K. J., Ngoyi, M. J., Suzuki, T., Wada, K. and Ikeda, S. (2020). Local Perspectives on Ebola during Its Tenth Outbreak in DR Congo: A Nationwide Qualitative Study. *PloS one* 15(10): e0241120. https://doi.org/10.1371/journal.pone.0241120.

147 Muzembo, B. A., Ntontolo, N. P., Ngatu, N. R., Khatiwada, J., Ngombe, K. L., Numbi, O. L., Nzaji, K. M., Maotela, K. J., Ngoyi, M. J., Suzuki, T., Wada, K. and Ikeda, S. (2020). Local Perspectives on Ebola during Its Tenth Outbreak in DR Congo: A Nationwide Qualitative Study. *PloS one* 15(10): e0241120. https://doi.org/10.1371/journal.pone.0241120.

148 Ziv, Oren (2020). If Pandemic Hits, Unrecognized Bedouin Villages could 'become like northern Italy'. +972 Magazine, 29 March. https://www.972mag.com/coronavirus-unrecognized-bedouin-villages/ (accessed 24 June 2020).

149 Nasser, Makbula (2020). 'A glimpse into the chaos': How Israel's COVID-19 Policy Neglects Palestinian Citizens. +972 Magazine, 21 September. https://www.972mag.com/palestinian-citizens-arabic-israel-coronavirus/ (accessed 20 January 2021).

150 Levy, Gideon and levac, Alex (2017). The Miraculous Tale of the West Bank's First University Hospital and Its 'Very Israeli' CEO. *Haaretz*, 19 August.

151 Reuters (2018). Trump Cuts $25 Million in Aid for Palestinians in East Jerusalem hospitals, 08 September. https://www.reuters.com/article/us-usa-palestinians-hospitals-idUSKCN1LO0O0 (accessed 20 February 2020).

152 Medical Aid for Palestinians (MAP) (2021). Three Palestinian Hospitals Attacked in Less than a Month Amid Global Pandemic, 22 January. https://www.map.org.uk/news/archive/post/1189-three-palestinian-hospitals-attacked-in-less-than-a-month-amid-global-pandemic (accessed 16 May 2021).

153 McNeely, C. A., Barber, B. K., Giacaman, R., Belli, R. F. and Daher, M. (2018). Long-Term Health Consequences of Movement Restrictions for Palestinians, 1987-2011. *American Journal of Public Health* 108(1): 77–83. https://doi.org/10.2105/AJPH.2017.304043.

Chapter 2

1 Lustick, Ian (2019). *Paradigm Lost: From Two-State Solution to One-State Reality*. Philadelphia: Pennsylvania University Press.

2 Suárez, Thomas (2017). *State of Terror: How Terrorism Created Modern Israel*. Northampton: Olive Branch Press. Piterberg, Gabriel (2008). *The Returns of Zionism: Myths, Politics and Scholarship in Israel*. London: Verso.

3 Masalha, Nur (2002). The Palestinian Nakba: Zionism, 'Transfer' and the 1948 Exodus. *Global Dialogue* 4 (Summer): 3; ProQuest Business Collection. See also, Sayegh, Fayez (1965). *Zionist Colonialism in Palestine*. Beirut: Research Center, Palestine Liberation Organization.

4 Wolfe, Patrick (2006). Settler Colonialism and the Elimination of the Native. *Journal of Genocide Research* 8(4): 388–9.

5 Pappé, I. and Chomsky, N. (2015). *On Palestine*. Haymarket Books.

6 Sharon Maintains Control in Face of Demographic Shift. *The Irish Times*, 20 August 2005. https://www.irishtimes.com/opinion/sharon-maintains -control-in-face-of-demographic-shift-1.482484 (accessed 18 June 2020).

7 Ophir, Adi (2007). There Are No Tortures in Gaza. *South Central Review* 24: 33.

8 Veracini, Lorenzo (2010). *Settler Colonialism: A Theoretical Overview*. Basingstoke: Palgrave Macmillan.

9 Gisha, Legal Center for Freedom of Movement (2018). Gaza Access and Movement: 2018 Summary. https://www.gisha.org/UserFiles/ File/publications/Gaza_Access_and_Movement_2018_Summary.pdf (accessed 07 June 2021).

10 Melon, Mercedes (2011). Shifting Paradigms, Israel's Enforcement of the Buffer Zone in the Gaza Strip.

11 Haddad, Toufic (2016). *Palestine Ltd: Neoliberalism and Nationalism in the Occupied Territories*. London: I.B. Taurus; Bouillon, Markus

E. (2004). Gramsci, Political Economy, and the Decline of the Peace Process. *Critique: Critical Journal of Middle East Studies* 13, no. 3 (Fall): 239–64; Bouris, Dimitris (2010). The European Union's Role in the Palestinian Territory after the Oslo Accords: Stillborn State-Building. *Journal of Contemporary European Research* 6(3): 376–94. http://www .jcer.net/ojs/index.php/jcer/article/view/205/232 (20 July 2020).

12 Amnesty International UK (2017). Gaza: Operation 'Cast Lead', 16 February. https://www.amnesty.org.uk/gaza-operation-cast-lead#:~ :text=On%2027%20December%202008%20Israel,agencies%20from %20entering%20the%20area.&text=Palestinian%20armed%20groups %20killed%20thirteen,rocket%20attacks%20on%20Southern%20Israel.

13 Al-Haq (2013). Voices From the Gaza Strip: A Year After Operation 'Pillar of Defense', 21 November. https://www.alhaq.org/monitoring -documentation/6700.html (accessed 08 June 2020).

14 United Nations Office for the Coordination of Humanitarian Affairs (OCHA) (2015). Key Figures on the 2014 Hostilities, 23 June. https:// www.ochaopt.org/content/key-figures-2014-hostilities (accessed 08 June 2020).

15 United Nations Office for the Coordination of Humanitarian Affairs (UN-OCHA occupied Palestinian territory) (2014) Occupied Palestinian Territory: Gaza Emergency Situation, September (Online). https:// www.ochaopt.org/sites/default/files/ocha_opt_sitrep_04_09_2014.pdf (accessed 08 June 2020).

16 Mughrabi, Nidal, Saul, Jonathan and Ayyub, Rami (2021). Israel and Hamas Both Claim Victory as Ceasefire Holds. *Reuters*, 21 May. https:// www.reuters.com/world/middle-east/gaza-truce-between-israel-Hamas -begins-mediated-by-egypt-2021-05-20/ (accessed 14 June 2021).

17 Hass, Amira (2021). Gaza Lives Erased: Israel Is Wiping Out Entire Palestinian Families on Purpose. *Haaretz*, 19 May. https://www.haaretz .com/israel-news/gaza-israel-wiping-entire-palestinian-families-Hamas -1.9820005 (accessed 07 June 2021).

18 Cohen, Dan (2014). In the Last Days of 'Operation Protective Edge' Israel Focused on Its Final Goal – The Destruction of Gaza's Professional Class. Mondoweiss, 13 October. http://mondoweiss.net/2014/10/protective -destruction-professional (accessed 07 June 2021).

19 Lloyd, David (2012). Settler Colonialism and the State of Exception: The Example of Palestine/Israel. *Settler Colonial Studies* 2(1): 59–80.

20 Sayegh, Fayez (1965). *Zionist Colonialism in Palestine, 1965*. Beirut: Research Center, Palestine Liberation Organization.

21 FACTS Information Committee (1988). 'Towards a State of Independence: The Palestinian Uprising, December 1987–August 1988', 106. http://www.jmcc.org/Documentsandmaps.aspx?id=609 (accessed 07 September 2020).

22 Khalidi, Rashid (2013). *Brokers of Deceit: How the US has Undermined Peace in the Middle East*. Boston: Beacon Press.

23 Sayegh, F. (1979). The Camp David Agreement and the Palestine Problem. *Journal of Palestine Studies* 8(2): 3–40.

24 Also known as the Gaza–Jericho Agreement.

25 Roy, S. (2002). Why Peace Failed: An Oslo Autopsy. *Current History* 101(651): 8–16.

26 Aruri, Nasser (1999). The Wye Memorandum: Netanyahu's Oslo and Unreciprocal Reciprocity. *Journal of Palestine Studies* 25(2): 17–28.

27 Sayigh, Y. (2009). 'Fixing Broken Windows': Security Sector Reform in Palestine, Lebanon, and Yemen. *Carnegie Papers,* Washington: Carnegie Endowment for International Peace.

28 Roy, Sara (2002). Ending the Palestinian Economy. *Middle East Policy* 9(4): 122–65; Sayigh, Y. (2009). 'Fixing Broken Windows': Security Sector Reform in Palestine, Lebanon, and Yemen. *Carnegie papers,* Washington: Carnegie Endowment for International Peace; Savir, Uri (1998). *The Process: 1,100 Days that Changed the Middle East*. New York: Random House.

29 Savir, Uri (1998). *The Process: 1,100 Days that Changed the Middle East*. New York: Random House.

30 Fanon, Frantz (1963). *The Wretched of the Earth*. New York: Grove Press.

31 Hilal, Jamil (2015). Rethinking Palestine: Settler-Colonialism, Neoliberalism and Individualism in the West Bank and Gaza Strip. *Contemporary Arab Affairs*. doi: 10.1080/17550912.2015.1052226.

32 World Health Organization-Palestinian Occupied Territory (2022). COVID-19 Monthly Situation Report, February. http://www.emro.who .int/images/stories/palestine/documents/covid-19-sit-rep-february-2022 .pdf?ua=1 (accessed 05 August 2022).

33 Middle East Eye (2022). Israeli Forces Arrest Senior Islamic Jihad Leader in Raid that Kills Palestinian Youth, 01 August. https://www .middleeasteye.net/news/israeli-forces-arrest-senior-islamic-jihad-leader -raid-kills-palestinian-youth (15 September 2022).

34 Kingsley, Patrick (2022). Another Gaza Conflict, but with a Difference: Hamas Sat It Out. *The New York Times*, 8 August. https://www.nytimes.com/2022/08/08/world/middleeast/gaza-Hamas-israel-islamic-jihad.html (15 September 2022).

35 Palestinian Islamic Resistance Movement (Hamas) (2018). Hamas: Despite Our Right to Armed Struggle, We Chose Peaceful Means, 17 May. https://Hamas.ps/en/post/1327/Hamas-Despite-our-right-to-armed-struggle-we-chose-peaceful-means (accessed 20 January 2020).

36 Al-Mughrabi, Nidal and Lubell, Mayyan (2022). Israel and Palestinian Militants Declare Gaza Truce. *Reuters*, 9 August. https://www.reuters.com/world/middle-east/palestinian-rockets-reach-west-jerusalem-third-day-gaza-fighting-2022-08-07/ (15 September 2022).

37 OXFAM International (2022). Fears that Wheat Stocks could Run Out in the Occupied Palestinian Territory within Three Weeks, 11 April. https://www.oxfam.org/en/press-releases/fears-wheat-stocks-could-run-out-occupied-palestinian-territory-within-three-weeks (05 August 2022).

38 Yair Lapid, the Israeli prime minister, said: 'There is another way. We will know to defend ourselves against anyone who threatens us, but we also know to give work and a livelihood and dignified life to anyone who wants to live peacefully beside us.' See Harkov, Lahav (2022). Lapid to Palestinians in Gaza: Take Your Future in Your Own Hands. *The Jerusalem Post*, 8 August. https://www.jpost.com/israel-news/article-714217 (15 September 2022).

39 al-Hajjar, Mohammed and Hussaini, Maha (2021). Gaza's Main COVID-19 Lab Halts Tests after Israel Bombing, 17 May. https://www.middleeasteye.net/news/gaza-covid-ceases-operations-israel-strike (accessed 07 June 2021).

40 Trew, Bel (2021). Gaza Medical Services Impacted after Israeli Airstrikes Damage Clinics and Hospitals, Say Health Officials. *Independent*, 16 May. https://www.independent.co.uk/news/world/middle-east/gaza-israel-airstrikes-hospitals-medics-b1848377.html (accessed 07 June 2021).

41 Suleiman, Jamil (2021). As a Doctor in Gaza, these have been the Most Difficult Days of My Life. +972 Magazine, 18 May. https://www.972mag.com/gaza-doctor-airstrikes/?fbclid=IwAR0R2tw_N5T2jCzQbZSE1Uq NIcRlheOPd6zfYnnIXq2AeL0IDHMVWez74OQ (accessed 07 June 2021).

42 B'Tselem (2017). The Gaza Strip, 11 November. https://www.btselem.org/ gaza_strip (accessed 07 June 2021).

43 Salamanca, Omar Jabary (2011). Unplug and Play: Manufacturing Collapse in Gaza. *Human Geography* 4(1): 22–37.

44 Agamben, Giorgio (1998). *Homo Sacer: Sovereign Power and Bare Life*. Stanford: Stanford University Press.

45 Journal of Palestine Studies (2009). A Gaza Chronology, 1948–2008. *Journal of Palestine Studies* XXXVIII, no. 3 (Spring): 98–121.

46 Memmi, A. (1974). *The Colonizer and the Colonized*. London: Souvenir Press.

47 Hamas (*Harakat al-Muqawama al-Islamiyya fi Filastin*) was established in 1988, and its military wing (the Izzedin al-Qassam Brigades) was formed a year later. In the First *Intifada*, it repeatedly undermined the Palestinian national leadership's commitment to non-violent resistance. Israel responded by introducing a permit system for Palestinian workers in Israel and also tried to crush the group by applying physical force. General Amram Mitzna, head of Israeli central command in the First *Intifada*, acknowledged this was preferable to suppressing popular resistance (Naser-Najjab, 2020).

48 Naser-Najjab, Nadia (2020). Palestinian Leadership and the Contemporary Significance of the First Intifada. *Race & Class* 62(2): 61–79.

49 Naser-Najjab, Nadia and Khatib, Ghassan (2019). The First Intifada, Settler Colonialism and Contemporary Prospects for Collective Resistance. *The Middle East Journal* 73(2): 187–206.

50 Harkov, Lahav (2019). Netanyahu: Money to Hams Part of Strategy to Keep Palestinians Divided. *The Jerusalem Post*, 12 March. https://www .jpost.com/Arab-Israeli-Conflict/Netanyahu-Money-to-Hamas-part-of -strategy-to-keep-Palestinians-divided-583082 (accessed 02 August 2020).

51 Ahren, Rapheal (2014). Netanyahu: Abbas must choose between Israel and Hamas. *The Times of Israel*, 23 April. https://www.timesofisrael.com /netanyahu-abbas-must-choose-between-israel-and-Hamas/ (accessed 07 June 2021).

52 Roy, Sara (2017). If Israel were Smart. *London Review of Books* 39(12). Available at: https://www.lrb.co.uk/v39/n12/sara-roy/if-israel-were -smart (accessed 07 June 2021).

Tibon, Amir (2018). Trump Administration Released Dozens of Millions of Dollars to Support Palestinian Security Forces. *Haartetz*, 2 August. https://www.haaretz.com/us-news/.premium-trump -administration-released-dozens-of-millions-of-dollars-to-pa-1.6340023 (accessed 07 June 2021).

53 Abdeen, Isam (2018). Legal Implications of Salary Cuts by the Palestinian Authority in the Gaza Strip. *Al-Haq*, 14 May. Legal Implications of Salary Cuts by the Palestinian Authority in the Gaza Strip (alhaq.org).

54 Swisher, Clayton E. (2011). *The Palestine Papers: The End of the Road.* London: Hesperus Press Limited.

55 Lazaroff, Tovah (2021). Israel Debates Banning COVID-19 vaccines for Gaza until Captives Released. *The Jerusalem Post*, 15 February. https:// www.jpost.com/arab-israeli-conflict/israel-debates-linking-covid-19 -vaccines-for-gaza-with-captive-release-659066 (accessed 07 June 2021).

56 Salamanca, Omar Jabary (2011). Unplug and Play: Manufacturing Collapse in Gaza. *Human Geography* 4(1): 22–37.

57 Badarin, E. (2016). *Palestinian Political Discourse: Between Exile and Occupation.* London: Routledge, 159.

58 Mbembe, A. (2003). Necropolitics. *Public Culture* 15(3): 11–40.

59 Mbembe, A. (2003). Necropolitics. *Public Culture* 15(3): 11–40.

60 United Nations Office for the Coordination of Humanitarian Affairs (OCHA) (2013). Access Restricted Areas (ARA) in the Gaza Strip. https://www.ochaopt.org/sites/default/files/ocha_opt_gaza_ara_factsheet _july_2013_english.pdf (accessed 07 June 2021).

61 B'Tselem (2020). Summer 2020: Gaza's Electricity Crisis Deepens Again, with 4 Hours of Daily Supply, 29 October. https://www.btselem.org/ gaza_strip/20201029_gaza_electricity_crisis_deepens_summer_2020 (accessed 07 June 2021).

62 Fanon, Frantz (1994). *A Dying Colonialism.* Boston: Grove Atlantic.

63 Abujidi, Nurhan (2009). The Palestinian States of Exception and Agamben. *Contemporary Arab Affairs* 2(2): 272–91.

64 Fanon, Frantz (1963). *The Wretched of the Earth.* New York: Grove Press.

65 Fanon, Frantz (1963). *The Wretched of the Earth.* New York: Grove Press.

66 Gisha (2017). The Dual Use List Finally Gets Published but it's the Opposite of Useful, 20 April. https://gisha.org/en-blog/2017/04/20/the -dual-use-list-finally-gets-published-but-its-the-opposite-of-useful/

67 Gisha (2012). Reader: 'Food Consumption in the Gaza Strip - Red Lines'. https://www.gisha.org/UserFiles/File/publications/redlines/redlines -position-paper-eng.pdf (accessed 07 June 2021).

68 Reuters (2011). Israel Said Would Keep Gaza Near Collapse: WikiLeaks, 5 January. https://www.reuters.com/article/us-palestinians-israel -wikileaks-idUSTRE7041GH20110105 (accessed 07 June 2021).

69 Mbembe, A. (2003). Necropolitics. *Public Culture* 15(3): 11–40.

70 Winter, Yves (2016). The Siege of Gaza: Spatial Violence, Humanitarian Strategies, and the Biopolitics of Punishment. *Constellations* 23(2): 308–19.

71 Winter, Yves (2016). The Siege of Gaza: Spatial Violence, Humanitarian Strategies, and the Biopolitics of Punishment. *Constellations* 23(2): 308–19.

72 Winter, Yves (2016). The Siege of Gaza: Spatial Violence, Humanitarian Strategies, and the Biopolitics of Punishment. *Constellations* 23(2): 308–19.

73 Abu-Sittah, G. (2020). The Virus, the Settler, and the Siege: Gaza in the Age of Corona. *Journal of Palestine Studies* 49(4): 65–76.

74 Abu-Sittah, G. (2020). The Virus, the Settler, and the Siege: Gaza in the Age of Corona. *Journal of Palestine Studies* 49(4): 65–76.

75 Medical Aid for Palestinians (MAP) (2022). Delayed, Denied and Deprived: The Collective Punishment of Palestinian Patients in Gaza in the Context of Israel's 15-Year Blockade, June. https://www.map.org .uk/downloads/map-al-mezan-access-to-health-online.pdf (accessed 15 September 2022).

76 Abunimah, Ali (2013). New UK Drones 'Field Tested' on Captive Palestinians. *Electronic Intifada*, 13 December. http://electronicintifada .net/blogs/ali-abunimah/new-uk-dronesfield-tested-captive-palestinians.

77 Hever, Shir (2017). *The Privatization of Israeli Security*. London: Pluto Press.

78 Sherwood, Harriet (2013). Israel Is World's Largest Drone Exporter. *The Guardian*, 20 May. https://www.theguardian.com/world/2013/may/20/ israel-worlds-largest-drone-exporter.

79 The United Nations Country Team in the Occupied Territory (2017). Gaza Ten Years Later, July. https://unsco.unmissions.org/sites/default/ files/gaza_10_years_later_-_11_july_2017.pdf (accessed 20 May 2021).

80 Fatma Ashour, a lawyer and writer from Gaza, posted on Facebook, during
the May 2021 war in the Strip. It is worthwhile to quote her post in full:

Unrevealed humanitarian cases during the current aggression in Gaza:
These cases are not neglected, but rather undisclosed due to the horror
we are going through, and therefore we hope that stakeholders could
help whenever they can.

* I received an appeal from a woman who has been suffering of
domestic violence since the beginning of the war. She was able to flee
at last, but she could not find a shelter, so she returned to her abusive
husband's house.

* It is extremely difficult for the elderly to move at a time when homes
are threatened, especially the disabled.

* Corona cases are not discovered in wartime after the bombing of the
only clinic that examines corona in Gaza.

* A number of women miscarried their babies out of fear.

* Those who have children suffering from autism and difficulty dealing
with them.

* Some children started hurting themselves, biting their hands and feet.

* There is extreme danger threatens to the lives of cancer patients due
to the lack of medicine and the date of their treatment is overdue.

* Concerned about the obsession of the high school students after the
Ministry of Education announced that the dates of the examinations as
they are.

* It is extremely dangerous to the life of those who have high blood
pressure and diabetes and have had previous strokes.

* Single mothers who do not have any money to buy their needs and
cannot move due to the danger of leaving the house and their inability
to leave their children alone.

There are dozens of unspoken needs that need to be solved

Please share, publish and help those vulnerable People. Fatma Ashour
(19 May 2021).

81 Monthly Humanitarian Bulletin: May 2018, UN OCHA OPT, 5 June
2018. https://www.ochaopt.org/content/monthly-humanitarian-bulletin
-may-2018 (accessed 23 May 2021).

82 Amjad Yaghi, a young freelance journalist in Gaza. Zoom interview, 10 June 2021.

83 Yara, not her real name, an activist, resident of Gaza. WhatsApp conversation, 28 May 2021.

84 Dr. Yehia Abed, Yehia Abed MD, MPH, Dr.PH, Al Quds University, School of Public Health, Gaza City, Gaza, WhatsApp conversation, 11 May 2021.

85 Interview, Rawia Hamam, director of training and scientific research department at Gaza Community Mental Health Programme – GCMHP, Messenger conversation, 05 May 2021.

86 Interview, Rawia Hamam, director of training and scientific research department at Gaza Community Mental Health Programme – GCMHP, Messenger conversation, 05 May 2021.

87 Middle East Monitor. Egypt Mediators to Visit West Bank, Gaza Strip Next Week, 15 August 2020. https://www.middleeastmonitor.com /20200815-egypt-mediators-to-visit-west-bank-gaza-strip-next-week/ (accessed 20 May 2021).

88 Interview, Ahmad, not his real name, in the field of nursing and psychology, Gaza. Messenger conversation, 03 May 2021.

89 United Nations Office for the Coordination of Humanitarian Affairs (OCHA) (2020a). Two Years On: People Injured and Traumatized During 'Great March of Return' Still Struggling, 6 April. https://www .ochaopt.org/content/two-years-people-injured-and-traumatized-during -great-march-return-are-stillstruggling#ftn3 (accessed 20 May 2021). (see also Amnesty International UK (2018). Israel: 'Deliberate Attempts' by Military to Kill and Maim Gaza Protesters Continues, 27 April 2018. https://www.amnesty.org.uk/press-releases/israel-deliberate-attempts -military-kill-and-maim-gaza-protesters-continues (accessed 20 May 2021).

90 Glazer, Hilo (2020). '42 Knees in One Day': Israeli Snipers Open Up About Shooting Gaza Protesters. *Haaretz*, 06 May. https://www.haaretz .com/israel-news/.premium.HIGHLIGHT.MAGAZINE-42-knees-in-one -day-israeli-snipers-open-up-about-shooting-gaza-protesters-1.8632555 (accessed 20 May 2021).

91 Puar, Jasbir K. (2015). The 'Right' to Maim: Disablement and Inhumanist Biopolitics in Palestine. *Borderlands* 14(1): 8.

92 Al Jazeera (2021). *Gaza Sees Spike in Coronavirus Cases: Health Ministry*, 31 March. https://www.aljazeera.com/news/2021/3/31/gaza-sees-spike-in-coronavirus-cases?fbclid=IwAR0_0UGCWBBtmWXldjR7I8rQRMn3KAh8Yi7xBeAI6fc5Xh2iNq7P_Q-vRWU (accessed 20 May 2021).

93 Lina, not her real name, health professional and researcher, Messenger conversation, 02 May 2021.

94 Al Mezan Center For Human Rights (2021). *Press Release: Al Mezan Condemns Israel's Blocking of COVID-19 Vaccine to Gaza*, 16 February. http://www.mezan.org/en/post/23917/Press+Release%3A+Al+Mezan+condemns+Israel%E2%80%99s+blocking+of+COVID-19+vaccine+to+Gaza+ (accessed 20 May 2021).

95 United Nations Office for the Coordination of Humanitarian Affairs (OCHA) (2020). *Deterioration in the Mental Health Situation in the Gaza Strip*, 05 October. https://www.ochaopt.org/content/deterioration-mental-health-situation-gaza-strip.

96 Medical Aid for Palestinians (MAP) (2017). *COVID-19 Cases Double again in Palestine: MAP Response Continues*, 10 July. https://www.map.org.uk/news/archive/post/1134-covid-19-cases-double-again-in-palestine-map-response-continues.

97 Lina, not her real name, health professional and researcher, Messenger conversation, 02 May 2021.

98 Interview, Rawia Hamam, director of training and scientific research department at Gaza Community Mental Health Programme – GCMHP, Messenger conversation, 05 May 2021.

99 Interview, Rawia Hamam, director of training and scientific research department at Gaza Community Mental Health Programme – GCMHP, Messenger conversation, 05 May 2021.

100 Saleh Abu Shamala, Youth Policy Club coordinator and researcher at Civitas Institute, Zoom meeting, 05 June 2021.

101 Interview, Rawia Hamam, director of training and scientific research department at Gaza Community Mental Health Programme – GCMHP, Messenger conversation, 05 May 2021.

102 The UN agency serves 70 per cent of refugees in the Strip, who account for 1.6 million of the Strip's two million inhabitants. They are corralled into 365 square kilometres.

103 The United Nations Relief and Works Agency for Palestine Refugees in the Near East (UNRWA) (2013). Gaza in 2020: UNRWA Operational Response May 2013 – Report, May. https://www.un.org/unispal/document/auto-insert-197872/ (accessed 20 May 2021).

104 Abed, Y. (2020). COVID-19 in the Gaza Strip and the West Bank under the Political Conflict in Palestine. *South Eastern European Journal of Public Health (SEEJPH)* XIV: 1–12. doi: 10.4119/seejph-3543.

105 United Nations General Assembly. Economic Costs of the Israeli Occupation for the Palestinian People: The Gaza Strip under Closure and Restrictions, 13 August 2020. https://unctad.org/system/files/official-document/a75d310_en_1.pdf (accessed 08 June 2021).

106 Alkhaldi, M. (2020). Health System's Response to the COVID-19 Pandemic in Conflict Settings: Policy Reflections from Palestine. *Global Public Health* 15(8): 1244–56.

107 B'Tselem (2021). Since Pandemic, has Israel Allowed almost no Palestinians Out of Gaza for Medical Treatment, 03 May. https://www.btselem.org/gaza_strip/20210503_gaza_patients_denied_treatment_since_covid_19_outbreak (accessed 09 August 2021).

108 Help Age International (2020). Gaza: Thousands of Lives of Chronic Disease Patients at Risk during COVID-19 Pandemic, 23 June. https://www.helpage.org/newsroom/latest-news/gaza-thousands-of-lives-of-chronic-disease-patients-at-risk-during-covid19-pandemic/ (accessed 20 July 2020).

109 Gisha (2011). Scale of Control: Israel's Continued Responsibility in the Gaza Strip, November. http://gisha.org/UserFiles/File/scaleofcontrol/scaleofcontrol_en.pdf (accessed 11 June 2021).

110 The Electronic Intifada (2008). Israel Continues to Coerce Gaza Patients into Collaboration. Al Mezan Center For Human Rights, 12 November. https://electronicintifada.net/content/israel-continues-coerce-gaza-patients-collaboration/868 (12 June 2021).

111 Tawil-Souri, Helga (2012). Digital Occupation: Gaza's High-Tech Enclosure. *Journal of Palestine Studies* 41, no. 2(Winter): 27–43.

112 Office for the Coordination of Humanitarian Affairs (OCHA) (2019). Gaza Strip Hospitals and Clinics, December 2018, 18 March. https://www.un.org/unispal/wp-content/uploads/2019/09/OCHAGAZAHOS_180319.pdf (12 June 2021).

113 Mahmoud, Walid (2020). Gaza Declares COVID-19 Disaster with Health System Near Collapse. *Al Jazeera*, 23 November. https://www.aljazeera .com/news/2020/11/23/gaza-declares-covid-19-disaster-with-health -system-near-collapse (accessed 12 June 2021).

114 Occupied Palestinian Territory: Gaza Emergency Situation Repost (as of 4 September 2014), OCHA. http://unispal.un.org/UNISPAL.NSF/0/901 64F24E91DC62A85257D490067170F (accessed 12 June 2021).

115 B'Tselem (2019). The Israeli Information Center for Human Rights in the Occupied Territories. 4.5 Years After Israel Destroyed Thousands of Homes in Operation Protective Edge: 13,000 Gazans Still Homeless. B'Tselem. https://www.btselem.org/gaza_strip/20190303_13000_gazans _homelsess_since_2014_war (accessed 12 June 2021).

116 Al Mezan Center for Human Rights (Al Mezan), Lawyers for Palestinian Human Rights (LPHR), and Medical Aid for Palestinians (MAP) (2020). Chronic Impunity for Attacks is Keeping Palestinian Health Workers in the Firing Line, 30 March. https://www.map.org.uk/downloads/chronic -impunity-gazas-health-sector-under-repeated-attack.pdf (accessed 12 June 2021).

117 Dr Yehia Abed, WhatsApp conversation, 11 May 2021.

118 Abu-Odah, H., Ramazanu, S., Saleh, E., Bayuo, J., Abed, Y. and Salah, M. S. (2021). COVID-19 Pandemic in Hong Kong and Gaza Strip: Lessons Learned from Two Densely Populated Locations in the World. *Osong Public Health Res Perspect* 12(1): 44–50. doi: 10.24171/j. phrp.2021.12.1.07. PMID: 33659154; PMCID: PMC7899229.

119 The Palestine–Turkey Friendship Hospital was established at the end of March 2020. It was donated by Turkey to help the PA combat COVID-19 (see OCHA-Relief Web, 2021). OCHA-Relief Web (2021). The Hospital Built by TİKA Reduces the Burden of COVID19 in Gaza, 14 April. The Hospital Built by TİKA Reduces the Burden of COVID19 in Gaza – occupied Palestinian territory | ReliefWeb (accessed 06 May 2021).

120 Abu-Odah, H., Ramazanu, S., Saleh, E., Bayuo, J., Abed, Y. and Salah, M. S. (2021). COVID-19 Pandemic in Hong Kong and Gaza Strip: Lessons Learned from Two Densely Populated Locations in the World. *Osong Public Health Res Perspect* 12(1): 44–50. doi: 10.24171/j. phrp.2021.12.1.07. PMID: 33659154; PMCID: PMC7899229.

121 Ahmad, not his real name, in the field of nursing and psychology, Gaza. Messenger conversation, 03 May 2021. Messenger conversation, 03 May 2021; Yara, not her real name, an activist, resident of Gaza. WhatsApp conversation 28 May 2021.

122 Ahmad, not his real name, in the field of nursing and psychology, Gaza. Messenger conversation, 03 May 2021.

123 Mohamed Ramadan, Monitoring and Evaluation Consultant, UNFPA (United Nations Fund for Population Activities), 10 May 2021.

124 Interview, Rawia Hamam, director of training and scientific research department at Gaza Community Mental Health Programme – GCMHP, Messenger conversation, 05 May 2021.

125 Akram, Fares (2019). Rare Protests Erupt against Hamas' 12-Year Rule over Gaza. *Associated Press*, 19 March. https://apnews.com/article/blockades-gaza-strip-israel-middle-east-arrests-8fdc192372ed472d804 3498f077d1dc0 (accessed 02 June 2021).

126 Interview, Ahmad, not his real name, in the field of nursing and psychology, Gaza. Messenger conversation, 03 May 2021.

127 Rettman, Adrew (2012). Hamas Appeals for Talks with EU Diplomats. *Euro Observer*, 03 December. https://euobserver.com/foreign/118392 (accessed 20 June 2021).

128 The Guardian (2013). Hamas Claims Increased Contact with European Countries, 12 July. https://www.theguardian.com/world/2013/jul/12/european-Hamas-contact-eu-gaza (20 June 2021).

129 The Guardian (2021). EU Sidelined and Divided as War Rages again in Middle East, 18 May. https://www.theguardian.com/world/2021/may/18/eu-sidelined-and-divided-as-war-rages-again-in-middle-east (accessed 09 June 2021).

130 Middle East Eye (2021). Israel-Palestine: Qatar Announces $500m for Gaza Reconstruction, 27 May. https://www.middleeasteye.net/news/israel-palestine-qatar-gaza-aid-reconstruction (accessed 08 September 2021).

131 MIFTAH (2012). Hamas Corruption Weighs Heavily on Gaza, 01 October. http://miftah.org/Display.cfm?DocId=25318&CategoryId=5 (20 June 2021).

132 Schoeberlein, Jennifer (2019). Transparency International Anti-Corruption Brief. Corruption in the Middle East & North Africa,

10 December. https://www.transparency.org/files/content/pages/2019
_GCB_MENA_country_profiles.pdf (accessed 09 August 2021).

133 Amnesty International (2019). Gaza: Journalist Facing Prison Term
for Exposing Corruption in Hamas-Controlled Ministry, 25 February.
https://www.amnesty.org/en/latest/news/2019/02/gaza-journalist-facing
-prison-term-for-exposing-corruption-in-Hamas-controlled-ministry/
(accessed 08 June 2021).

134 Saleh Abu Shamala, Youth Policy Club coordinator and researcher at
Civitas Institute, Zoom meeting, 05 June 2021.

135 Al Haq (2019). Q&A The Great Return March: One Year On, 25 May.
https://www.alhaq.org/advocacy/6044.html (accessed 09 June 2021).

136 Aid from Qatar in 2019 to help Palestinians in the occupied territory.
A three days of Israeli air strikes on Gaza and Hamas rockets at Israel
ended by reaching a ceasefire in May 2019. Following the ceasefire Qater
pledged to send money for humanitarian and economic aid.

137 Ynet News (2019). 'Where's the Qatari Money?' Hamas Facing Growing
Criticism in Gaza, 10 March. https://www.ynetnews.com/articles/0,7340
,L-5601366,00.html (accessed 21 July 2021).

138 Lina, not her real name, health professional and researcher, Messenger
conversation, 02 May 2021.

139 Clarno, Andy (2017). *Neoliberal Apartheid: Palestine/Israel and South
Africa after 1994*. Chicago and London: University of Chicago Press.

140 Farraj, Lamees and Dana, Tariq (2021). The Politicization of Public
Sector Employment and Salaries in the West Bank and Gaza. *Al Shabaka*,
14 March. https://al-shabaka.org/briefs/the-politicization-of-public
-sector-employment-and-salaries-in-palestine/ (accessed 21 July 2021).

141 Lazaroff, Tovah (2013). Gaza Officials Who do not Work Are Receiving
EU Paychecks. *The Jerusalem Post*, 11 December. https://www.jpost.com/
middle-east/gaza-officials-who-do-not-work-are-receiving-eu-paychecks
-334688 (accessed 21 July 2021).

142 Barzak, Ibrahim (2013). Audit: EU Pays Palestinians in Gaza Who Don't
Work. *AP News*, 11 December. https://apnews.com/article/6d605ed48f4
54295b4d9a1f30ae58ad1 (accessed 21 July 2021).

143 Hanieh, Adam (2008). Palestine in the Middle East: Opposing
Neoliberalism and US Power. *MRzine*, 19 July. http://www
.monthlyreview.org/mrzine; Hanieh, Lineages of Revolt

144 Abdeen, Isam (2018). Legal Implications of Salary Cuts by the Palestinian Authority in the Gaza Strip. *Al Haq*, 14 May. https://www.alhaq.org/advocacy/6220.html (accessed 20 July 2021).

145 Reuters (2020). Civil Servants to Receive only 50 percent of June Salary, 26 July. https://english.wafa.ps/Pages/Details/118657 (accessed 20 July 2021).

146 Interview, Ahmad, not his real name, in the field of nursing and psychology, Gaza. Messenger conversation, 03 May 2021.

147 Mohamed Ramadan, Monitoring and Evaluation Consultant, UNFPA (United Nations Fund for Population Activities), 10 May 2021.

148 Almasri, Abier (2017). In Gaza, We Get Four Hours of Electricity a Day — If We're Lucky. *Human Rights Watch*, 20 August. https://www.hrw.org/news/2017/08/20/gaza-we-get-four-hours-electricity-day-if-were-lucky (accessed 20 July 2021).

149 Mohamed Ramadan, Monitoring and Evaluation Consultant, UNFPA (United Nations Fund for Population Activities), 10 May 2021.

150 Yara, not her real name, an activist, resident of Gaza. WhatsApp conversation, 28 May 2021.

151 Haddad, Tamir (2012). Hamas Corruption Weighs Heavily on Gaza. MIFTAH, 01 October. http://miftah.org/Display.cfm?DocId=25318&CategoryId=5 (accessed 20 June 2021).

152 Fast, Larissa (2006). 'Aid in the Pressure Cooker' Humanitarian Action in the Occupied Palestinian Territory. *Humanitarian Agenda*, Case Study no. 7, Feinstein International Center, November 2006.

153 NGO Monitor (2020). In a First, EU to Investigate if Funding Went to Terror Linked NGOs, 20 May. https://www.ngo-monitor.org/eu-to-investigate-funding-terror-linked-ngos/ (accessed 19 September 2020).

154 Dr. Yehia Abed, Yehia Abed MD, MPH, Dr.PH, Al Quds University, School of Public Health, Gaza City, Gaza, WhatsApp conversation, 11 May 2021.

155 Dr. Yehia Abed, Yehia Abed MD, MPH, Dr.PH, Al Quds University, School of Public Health, Gaza City, Gaza, WhatsApp conversation, 11 May 2021.

156 The Palestine Forum, which was created on 10 April 2018, includes a broad range of participants (Palestinian artists and activists, academics and intellectuals drawn) from historical Palestine, the oPt and the

diaspora. It organizes workshops and seminars and invites speakers to exchange ideas on how Palestinian institutions can be rebuilt and solutions can be developed. I became a member of the Forum's coordinating and intellectual committees at the end of 2020.

157 United Nations Office for the Coordination of Humanitarian Affairs (OCHA) (2021). Response to the Escalation in the oPt | Situation Report No. 1, 21–27 May 2021, 27 May. https://www.ochaopt.org/content/response-escalation-opt-situation-report-no-1-21-27-may-2021 (accessed 31 May 2021).

158 The World Bank (2017). Reconstructing Gaza - Donor Pledges, 12 September. https://www.worldbank.org/en/programs/rebuilding-gaza-donor-pledges (accessed 31 May 2021).

159 Wolfe, Patrick (2006). Settler Colonialism and the Elimination of the Native. *Journal of Genocide Research* 8(4): 388–9.

Chapter 3

1 Palestinian Central Bureau of Statistics. http://www.pcbs.gov.ps/Portals/_Rainbow/Documents/HebronE.html.

2 B'Tselem (2007). Ghost Town: Israel's Separation Policy and Forced Eviction of Palestinians from the Center of Hebron. Publications. http://www.btselem.org/publications/summaries/200705_hebron (accessed 09 June 2021). Shalhoub-Kevorkian, N. (2015). *Security Theology, Surveillance and the Politics of Fear.* Cambridge Studies in Law and Society, Cambridge: Cambridge University Press.

3 At the end of 2019, the US Secretary of State Mike Pompeo suggested 'the establishment of Israeli civilian settlements in the West Bank is not, per se, inconsistent with international law'. In response, Naftali Bennett, the Israeli defence minister, announced a plan to double the number of settlers in the heart of the city. See BBC News. US Says Israeli Settlements Are no Longer Illegal, 18 November 2019. https://www.bbc.co.uk/news/world-middle-east-50468025 (accessed 18 June 2021); Al Jazeera. Israel Planning New Settlement in Flashpoint City of Hebron, 15 January 2019. https://www.aljazeera.com/news/2019/12/1/israel-planning-new-settlement-in-flashpoint-city-of-hebron.

4 The New York Times (1973). Israel Expands Town In Occupied Territory, 28 June. https://www.nytimes.com/1973/06/28/archives/israel-expands -town-in-occupied-territory-emotion-and-politics.html (accessed 11 June 2021).

5 Peace Now (2016). Secret Document Reveals Settlements were Built on a Lie, 28 July. https://peacenow.org.il/en/kiryat-arba-seizuer (accessed 11 June 2021).

6 Dearden, Lizzie (2006). Secret 1970 Document Shows First Israeli Settlements in West Bank were Built under False Pretences. *Independent*, 30 July. Secret 1970 document shows first Israeli settlements in West Bank were built under false pretences | The Independent | The Independent (accessed 18 June 2021).

7 Shlaim, Avi (2000). *The Iron Wall: Israel and the Arab World*. London: Allen Lane, The Penguin Press.

8 Shlaim, Avi (2000). *The Iron Wall: Israel and the Arab World*. London: Allen Lane, The Penguin Press.

9 Raz, Avi (2021). *The Bride and the Dowry: Israel, Jordan and the Palestinians in the Aftermath of the June 1967 War*. New Haven: Yale University Press.

10 Weizman, Eyal (2007). *Hollow Land: Israel's Architecture of Occupation*. London: Verso Books. Halper, J. (2015). *War against the People: Israel, the Palestinians and Global Pacification*. London: Pluto Press.

11 Peace Now (2019). Bennett Promotes New Settlement in Hebron's Wholesale Market, 1 December. https://peacenow.org.il/en/a-new -settlement-in-the-wholesale-market-of-hebron (accessed 20 January 2020).

12 Giovannetti, Megan (2019). 'They have punished the victims': Hebron Struggles 25 years after Ibrahimi Mosque Massacre. Middle East Eye, 25 February. https://www.middleeasteye.net/news/they-have-punished -victims-hebron-struggles-25-years-after-ibrahimi-mosque-massacre.

13 OCHA (2013). Humanitarian Monitor Monthly Report (February 2013), 10. Available at: https://www.ochaopt.org/documents/ocha_opt_the _humanitarian_monitor_2013_03_25_english.pdf (accessed 10 June 2021).

14 B'Tselem (2003). Hebron, Area H-2: Settlements Cause Mass Departure of Palestinians, August. https://www.btselem.org/publications/

summaries/200308_hebron_area_h2 (accessed 12 November 2022).

2014. http://www.hebronrc.ps/images/stories/MP%20English.pdf (accessed 15 June 2021).

15 B'Tselem (2019). New B'Tselem Report about the City of Hebron: Using Security Excuses, Israel has Managed to Forcibly Transfer Palestinian Residents of the City, 25 September. https://www.btselem.org/press _releases/20190925_playing_the_security_card (accessed 08 June 2021).

16 BADIL Resource Center for Palestinian Residency & Refugee Rights (2016). Forced Population Transfer: The Case of the Old City of Hebron. https://www.badil.org/phocadownloadpap/badil-new/publications/ research/working-papers/CaseStudyFPT-Hebron-Brief-Eng(Oct2016). pdf (accessed 26 July 2021).

17 Hebron Rehabilitation Committee (HRC). https://www.hebronrc.ps/ index.php/en/about-hrc/mission-and-objectives (accessed 11 June 2021).

18 Article 11 of the Hebron Protocol restricts Palestinian building plans by requiring coordination with Israel for:

1. The proposed construction of buildings above two floors (6 meters) within 50 meters of the external boundaries of the locations
2. The proposed construction of buildings above three floors (9 meters) between 50 and 100 meters of the external boundaries
3. The proposed construction of non-residential, non-commercial buildings within 100 meters of the external boundaries of the locations …(such as industrial factories) or buildings and institutions in which more that 50 persons are expected to gather together
4. The proposed construction of buildings above two floors (6 meters) within 50 meters from each side of the road (JPS, 1997: 135).

19 Mharib, 'Abd al-Hafiz (1971, March). ālḥmāṭsm wālṣqwr fy āsrāyl ['Hawks and Doves' in Israel]. *Shu'un Filastiniyyah* 1: 5–26.

20 In Hebron city, the security of 479 settlers is privileged over the right to existence of 154, 714 Palestinian residents (PASSIA, 2003).

21 Journal of Palestine Studies. The Hebron Protocol (1997). *Journal of Palestine Studies* 26(3): 131–45. doi: 10.2307/2538174.

22 B'Tselem (2019). Hebron City Center, 11 November (updated 26 May 2019). https://www.btselem.org/hebron (accessed 27 June 2021).

23 Dr Hazem Ashhab, MD, head of gastroenterology,·Al-Ahli Hospital. Member of National Committee for CORONA. Zoom interview, 11 June 2021.

24 Sayegh, Fayez (1965). *Zionist Colonialism in Palestine, 1965*. Beirut: Research Center, Palestine Liberation Organization.

25 The Hebron Protocol (1997). *Journal of Palestine Studies* 26(3): 131–45. doi: 10.2307/2538174.

26 Andoni, Lamis (1997). Redefining Oslo: Negotiating the Hebron Protocol. *Journal of Palestine Studies* 25(3): 17–30.

27 The Hebron Protocol (1997). *Journal of Palestine Studies* 26(3): 131–45. doi: 10.2307/2538174.

28 Andoni, Lamis (1997). Redefining Oslo: Negotiating the Hebron Protocol. *Journal of Palestine Studies* 25(3): 17–30.

29 The Hebron Protocol (1997). *Journal of Palestine Studies* 26(3): 131–45. doi: 10.2307/2538174.

30 Journal of Palestine Studies (1997). Special Document File. The Hebron Protocol 26, no. 3 (spring): 131–45.

31 Addameer (2015). Israeli Occupation Arrests 1,195 Palestinians and Issues 128 Administrative Detention Orders. http://www.addameer.org/news/addameer-israeli-occupation-arrests1195-palestinians-and-issues-128-administrative-detention (accessed 13 June 2021).

32 Al-Haq (2013). Israeli Military Arrests More than 20 Palestinian Children in Hebron. http://www.alhaq.org/documentation/weekly-focuses/691-israeli-military-arrests-more-than-20-palestinian-children-in-hebron (accessed 14 June 2021).

33 Agamben, G. (2005). *State of Exception*. Chicago: University of Chicago Press.

34 Foucault, Michel (1990). *The History of Sexuality, Vol. 1, An Introduction*. Translated by Robert Hurley. London: Penguin Books.

35 World Health Organisation (WHO) (2010). Occupied Palestinian Territory, November. http://www.emro.who.int/pdf/pse/palestine-infocus/abu-abed.pdf?ua=1 (accessed 09 June 2021).

36 Agamben, G. (1998). *Homo Sacer: Sovereign Power and Bare Life*. Stanford: Stanford University Press.

37 Mbembe, A. (2003). Necropolitics. *Public Culture* 15(1): 11–40.

38 Hebron Rehabilitation Committee (2016). Two Palestinians Killed in Tel Rumeida on 24 March. http://www.hebronrc.ps/index.php/en/news/2038-2038 (accessed 13 June 2021).

39 Amnesty International (2015). Israel/OPT: Investigate Apparent Extrajudicial Execution at Hebron Hospital. Available at: https://www

.amnesty.org/en/latest/news/2015/11/israel-opt-investigateapparent
-extrajudicial-execution-at-hebron-hospital/ (accessed 13 June 2021).

40 Breaking the Silence (2017). The High Command, Settler Influence on IDF Conduct in the West Bank. https://www.breakingthesilence.org.il /inside/wp-content/uploads/2018/03/THC_Eng_210318.pdf (accessed 28 June 2021).

41 'Breaking the Silence' was established by soldiers who served in Hebron, who wanted '[t]o boost public awareness . . . with the aim of giving the Israeli public access to the reality that exists only minutes away from their own homes, yet is rarely portrayed in the media'. See Breaking the Silence: http://www.breakingthesilence.org.il/about/organization (accessed 27 June 2021).

42 Breaking the Silence (2018). Occupying Hebron, Soldiers' Testimonies from Hebron 2011–2017, November. https://www.breakingthesilence .org.il/inside/wp-content/uploads/2018/11/OccupyingHebron-Eng.pdf (accessed 28 June 2021).

43 Fawaz Abu Aisheh, employee at the Municipality of Hebron, Messenger conversation, 15 June 2021.

44 Konrad, Edo (2018). Seven Hospitalized in Settler Attack on Hebron Activists. +972 Magazine, 28 December. https://www.972mag.com/seven -palestinians-hospitalized-settler-attack-hebron-activists/ (accessed 16 June 2021).

45 Palreports Khalil (2015). Infamous Settler Anat Cohen Attacking Internationals, 15 December. Available at https://www.youtube.com/ watch?v=RLGOGxvZHds (accessed 16 June 2021).

46 B'Tselem (2015). Footage from Hebron: Israeli Military Enables 5-day Settler Attack. Available at: http://www.btselem.org/settler_violence /20151020_5_days_of_settler_attacks_in_hebron (accessed 14 June 2021).

47 Peace Now (2019). Court Orders Eviction of Settlers from Bakri House in Hebron, 18 March. https://peacenow.org.il/en/court-orders-eviction -of-settlers-from-bakri-house-in-hebron#.XI9vyyRbGcc.twitter (accessed 27 June 2021).

48 B'Tselem (2007). Tel Rumeida, Hebron, 01 November. https://www .btselem.org/video/2008/11/tel-rumeida-hebron#full (accessed 25 June 2021).

49 Yesh Din, which was established in 2005, documents Israel's violations of Palestinian human rights in the West Bank.

50 Yesh Din Figures (2018). Ideologically Motivated Crime by Settlers in Hebron Gets Tailwind from Israeli Authorities, November 2018. https:// s3-eu-west-1.amazonaws.com/files.yesh-din.org/Hebron_ENG_Nov18 .pdf (accessed 17 August 2022).

51 Hamdan, A. (2020). Silent Displacement in Occupied Palestine: Hebron as a Case Study (Doctoral dissertation, University of Exeter). Unpublished, permission has been granted.

52 Hamdan, A. (2020). Silent Displacement in Occupied Palestine: Hebron as a Case Study (Doctoral dissertation, University of Exeter). Unpublished, permission has been granted.

53 B'Tselem (2007). Daily Attacks by Settlers on the Abu 'Ayesha Family, Tel Rumeida, Hebron, 04 January. https://www.btselem.org/testimonies /20070104_settlers_attack_the_abu_ayesha_family_daily (accessed 16 June 2021).

54 Nour Abu Aisha, merchant, Messenger conversation, 13 June 2021.

55 B'Tselem (2019). Playing the Security Card, Israeli Policy in Hebron as a Means to Effect Forcible Transfer of Local Palestinians, September. https://www.btselem.org/sites/default/files/publications/201909_playing _the_security_card_eng.pdf (accessed 22 June 2021).

56 Nour Abu Aisha, merchant, Messenger conversation, 13 June 2021.

57 Hamdan, A. (2020). Silent Displacement in Occupied Palestine: Hebron as a Case Study (Doctoral dissertation, University of Exeter). Unpublished, permission has been granted.

58 BADIL Resource Center for Palestinian Residency & Refugee Rights (2016). Forced Population transfer: The Case of the Old City of Hebron. Brief, October. https://www.badil.org/phocadownloadpap/badil-new /publications/research/working-papers/CaseStudyFPT-Hebron-Brief -Eng(Oct2016).pdf (accessed 13 June 2021).

59 BADIL Resource Center for Palestinian Residency & Refugee Rights (2016). Forced Population Transfer: The Case of the Old City of Hebron. Brief, October. https://www.badil.org/phocadownloadpap/badil-new /publications/research/working-papers/CaseStudyFPT-Hebron-Brief -Eng(Oct2016).pdf (accessed 13 June 2021).

60 B'Tselem (2015). New Restrictions on Movement in Hebron and Environs Disrupt Lives and Constitute Prohibited Collective Punishment. https://www.btselem.org/freedom_of_movement/20151105 _hebron_area

61 OCHA (2020). Dignity Denied: Life in the Settlement Area of Hebron city, 20 February. https://www.ochaopt.org/content/dignity-denied-life -settlement-area-hebron-city (accessed 18 June 2021).

62 BADIL Resource Center for Palestinian Residency & Refugee Rights (2016). Forced Population transfer: The Case of the Old City of Hebron. Brief, October. https://www.badil.org/phocadownloadpap/badil-new /publications/research/working-papers/CaseStudyFPT-Hebron-Brief -Eng(Oct2016).pdf (accessed 13 June 2021).

63 Halper, J. (2021). *Decolonising Israel, Liberating Palestine: Zionism, Settler Colonialism, and the Case for One Democratic State*. London: Pluto Press. Wolfe, P. (2006). Settler Colonialism and the Elimination of the Native. *Journal of Genocide Research* 8(4): 387–409.

64 Quray', Aḥmad (2005). *al-Riwāyah al-Filasṭīnīyah al-kāmilah lil-mufāwaḍāt: min Ūslū ilá Kharīṭat al-ṭarīq*. Vol. 1. Bayrūt: Mu'assasat al-Dirāsāt al-Filasṭīnīyah.

65 B'Tselem (2013). The South Hebron Hills, 01 January. https://www .btselem.org/south_hebron_hills (accessed 11 June 2021.

66 B'Tselem (2013). The South Hebron Hills, 01 January. https://www .btselem.org/south_hebron_hills (accessed 11 June 2021.

67 B'tselem (2013). The South Hebron Hills, 01 January. https://www .btselem.org/south_hebron_hills (accessed 27 June 2021).

68 Nassar, Tamara (2018). Israel 'drastically escalates' Destruction of EU-Funded Energy Projects. Electronic Intifada, 26 March. https:// electronicintifada.net/blogs/tamara-nassar/israel-drastically-escalates -destruction-eu-funded-energy-projects (accessed 11 June 2021).

69 The Brussels Times (2020). Israel slammed for Demolition of Belgian-Funded Palestinian Homes, 06 November. https://www.brusselstimes .com/belgium/139493/israel-slammed-for-demolition-of-belgian -funded-palestinian-homes-eu-foreign-affairs-united-nations-al-rakeez -occupied-west-bank-palestine-territories-israeli-army-displacement -children/ (accessed 27 June 2021).

70 OCHA (2020). COVID-19 Emergency Situation Report 13 (1–14 July 2020), 14 July. https://www.ochaopt.org/content/covid-19-emergency -situation-report-13.

71 Middle East Monitor (2020). Israel Soldiers Destroy Another Palestinian Coronavirus Testing Centre, 23 July. https://www.middleeastmonitor

.com/20200723-israel-soldiers-destroy-another-palestinian-coronavirus
-testing-centre/ (accessed 27 June 2021).

72 Amnesty International (2021). Israeli Army Shutdown of Health
Organization will have Catastrophic Consequences for Palestinian
Healthcare, 09 June. https://www.amnesty.org/en/latest/news/2021/06
/israeli-army-shutdown-of-health-organization-will-have-catastrophic
-consequences-for-palestinian-healthcare/?fbclid=IwAR323DhreQOx5
2WLkrdFKg77wehxJ9uXoIqigxImKRlhwU0F3Q7n8N9ocWY (accessed
26 June 2021).

73 Kuttab, Daoud (2017). Hebron: 20 Years of Apartheid and Oppression.
The New Arab, 17 January. https://english.alaraby.co.uk/opinion/hebron
-20-years-apartheid-and-oppression (accessed 27 June 2021).

74 Nour Abu Aisha, merchant, Messenger conversation, 13 June 2021.

75 Dr. Hazem Ashhab, MD, head of gastroenterology,·Al-Ahli Hospital.
Member of National Committee for CORONA. Zoom interview, 11 June
2021.

76 Dr. Hazem Ashhab, MD, head of gastroenterology,·Al-Ahli Hospital.
Member of National Committee for CORONA. Zoom interview, 11 June
2021.

77 Majed, not his real name, Messenger conversation, 24 June 2021.

78 Amnesty International UK (2021). Palestine: Activist Nizar Banat's Death
in Custody 'raises serious alarm', 24 June. https://www.amnesty.org.uk
/press-releases/palestine-activist-nizar-banats-death-custody-raises
-serious-alarm (accessed 24 June 2021).

79 Majed, not his real name, Messenger conversation, 24 June 2021.

80 Kuttab, Daoud (2017). Hebron: 20 Years of Apartheid and Oppression.
The New Arab, 17 January. https://english.alaraby.co.uk/opinion/hebron
-20-years-apartheid-and-oppression (accessed 27 June 2021).

81 Abu Amer, Adnan (2020). Fatah 'Monopolises' Emergency Committees in
the West Bank, Excludes Hamas, 05 May. https://www.middleeastmonitor
.com/20200505-fatah-monopolises-emergency-committees-in-the-west
-bank-excludes-Hamas/ (accessed 20 June 2021).

82 Manal, not her real name, resident of Tel Remeida, Messenger
conversation, 22 December 2021.

83 Fawaz Abu Aisheh, employee at the Municipality of Hebron, Messenger
conversation, 15 June 2021.

84 Dr. Hazem Ashhab, MD, head of gastroenterology,·Al-Ahli Hospital. Member of National Committee for CORONA. Zoom interview, 11 June 2021.

85 Fuad al-Amour, Messenger interview, 07 July 2021.

86 Manal, not her real name, resident of Tel Remeida, Messenger conversation, 22 December 2021.

87 Manal, not her real name, resident of Tel Remeida, Messenger conversation, 22 December 2021.

88 Fuad al-Amour. Messenger interview, 07 July 2021.

89 Manal, not her real name, resident of Tel Remeida, Messenger conversation, 22 December 2021.

90 Abu Amer, Adnan (2020). Fatah 'Monopolises' Emergency Committees in the West Bank, Excludes Hamas, 05 May. https://www .middleeastmonitor.com/20200505-fatah-monopolises-emergency -committees-in-the-west-bank-excludes-Hamas/ (accessed 20 June 2021).

91 Hever, Shir and Naser-Najjab, Nadia (2020). Cracks in Israel's Separation Wall and Netanyahu's Fragile Grip on Power. Middle East Eye, 19 August. https://www.middleeasteye.net/opinion/israel-netanyahu-separation -wall-power-cracks-fragile (accessed 14 June 2021).

92 Sharabati was an activist in the First *Intifada*. He currently coordinates the Hebron Defense Committee. Messenger conversation, 09 October 2020.

93 Palestine New Federations of Trade Unions Statement (2020). 'New Unions May 1 Statement', 1 May. https://www.stopthewall.org/2020/05 /01/new-unions-may-1-statement (accessed 27 June 2021).

94 Samour, S. (2020). Covid-19 and the Necroeconomy of Palestinian Labor in Israel. *Journal of Palestine Studies* 49(4): 53–64.

95 Samour, S. (2020). Covid-19 and the Necroeconomy of Palestinian Labor in Israel. *Journal of Palestine Studies* 49(4): 53–64.

96 Samour, S. (2020). Covid-19 and the Necroeconomy of Palestinian Labor in Israel. *Journal of Palestine Studies* 49(4): 53–64.

97 Palestine News and Information Agency, WAFA (2020). Palestinian Government to Pay Its Employees only 50 percent of their Monthly Salary – Finance Minister, 02 July. http://english.wafa.ps/page.aspx?id =QNqpd6a118623638661aQNqpd6 (accessed 16 June 2021).

98 Fawaz Abu Aisheh, employee at the Municipality of Hebron, Messenger conversation, 15 June 2021.

99 Manal, not her real name, resident of Tel Remeida, Messenger conversation, 22 December 2021.

100 Mbembe, A. (2003). Necropolitics. *Public Culture* 15(3): 11–40.

101 Nour Abu Aisha, merchant, Messenger conversation, 13June 2021.

102 Fawaz Abu Aisheh, employee at the Municipality of Hebron, Messenger conversation, 15 June 2021.

103 Manal, not her real name, resident of Tel Remeida, Messenger conversation, 22 December 2021.

104 Fuad al-Amour, Messenger interview, 07 July 2021.

105 Fuad al-Amour, Messenger interview, 07 July 2021. See Darweish, Marwan (2016). Israeli Peace and Solidarity Organizations. In Ozerdem, Alpaslan, Thiessen, Chuck and Qassoum, Mufid (eds), *Conflict Transformation and the Palestinians*. Florence: Taylor and Francis, chapter 13, 229–45.

106 Dr. Hazem Ashhab, MD, head of gastroenterology, Al-Ahli Hospital. Member of National Committee for CORONA. Zoom interview, 11 June 2021.

107 Shezaf, Hagar (2021). Masked Israelis Filmed Throwing Stones at Palestinians While Soldiers Stood By. *Israel News*, 27 June.

108 Fuad al-Amour. Messenger interview, 07 July 2021.

109 Alazzeh, Ala (2015). Seeking Popular Participation: Nostalgia for the First Intifada in the West Bank. *Settler Colonial Studies* 5(3).

Chapter 4

1 B'Tselem (2017). East Jerusalem, 11 November. https://www.btselem.org/jerusalem (accessed 19 June 2021).

2 Human Rights Watch (2021). A Threshold Crossed, Israeli Authorities and the Crimes of Apartheid and Persecution. israel_palestine0421_reportcover_8.5x11 (hrw.org).

3 HaMoKed and B'Tselem (1997). The Quiet Deportation: Revocation of Residency of East Jerusalem Palestinians.

4 B'Tselem (2017). East Jerusalem, 11 November. https://www.btselem.org/ jerusalem (accessed 18 July 2020).

5 Bishara, Marwan (2001). *Palestine/Israel: Peace or Apartheid: Prospects for Resolving the Conflict.* London: Zed Books.

6 Weizman, Eyal (2007). *Hollow Land: Israel's Architecture of Occupation.* London: Verso.

7 Weizman, Eyal (2007). *Hollow Land: Israel's Architecture of Occupation.* London: Verso.

8 Adukhater, Jalal (2011). Israel Censors Palestinian Textbooks in East Jerusalem. +972 Magazine, October. http://972mag.com/israeli -authorities-impose-censored-palestinian-textbooks-in-east-jerusalem /26137/.

9 Wilson, Nigel (2016). Israel Tells Palestinians: Our Textbooks or No Funding. *Al Jazeera*, 01 September. https://www.aljazeera.com/news /2016/9/1/israel-tells-palestinians-our-textbooks-or-no-funding (accessed 21 June 2021).

10 Sa'di, A. H. (2016). *Thorough Surveillance: The Genesis of Israeli Policies of Population Management, Surveillance and Political Control towards the Palestinian Minority.* Manchester: Manchester University Press.

11 Al Tahhan (2022). Zena Palestinian Schools in Jerusalem Strike over Israel-Imposed Books. *Al Jazeera*, 19 September. https://www.aljazeera .com/news/2022/9/19/jerusalem-palestinian-schools-strike-over-israeli -imposed-books (accessed 20 September 2022).

12 Grande, S. (2015). *Red Pedagogy: Native American Social and Political Thought.* USA: Rowman & Littlefield.

13 B'Tselem (2017). East Jerusalem, 11 November. https://www.btselem.org/ jerusalem (accessed 19 June 2021).

14 B'Tselem (2014). National Parks as Tool for Constraining Palestinian Neighborhoods in East Jerusalem, 16 September. https://www.btselem .org/jerusalem/national_parks (accessed 19 June 2021).

15 HaMoKed and B'Tselem (1997). The Quiet Deportation: Revocation of Residency of East Jerusalem Palestinians.

16 Al Shabaka (2017). Residency Revocation: Israel's Forcible Transfer of Palestinians from Jerusalem, 03 July. https://al-shabaka.org/releases/ residency-revocation-israels-forcible-transfer-palestinians-jerusalem/ (19 June 2021).

17 B'Tselem (2017). East Jerusalem, 11 November. https://www.btselem.org/jerusalem (accessed 19 June 2021).

18 Fanon, Frantz (1963). *The Wretched of the Earth*. New York: Grove Press.

19 Joronen, M. (2019). Negotiating Colonial Violence: Spaces of Precarisation in Palestine. *Antipode* 51(3): 838–57.

20 Veracini, Lorenzo (2010). *Settler Colonialism: A Theoretical Overview*. Basingstoke: Palgrave Macmillan.

21 Tanous, Osama (2020). When Pandemics Hit Militarized Urban Spaces. Rosa Luxemburg Stiftung Office of Palestine and Jordan, 21 May. https://www.rosalux.ps/?p=3066 (accessed 14 June 2021).

22 Hammoudeh, D., Hamayel, L. and Welchman, L. (2016). Beyond the Physicality of Space: East Jerusalem, Kufr 'Aqab, and the Politics of Everyday Suffering. *The Jerusalem Quarterly* 65: 35–60.

23 Mbembe, A. (2003). Necropolitics. *Public Culture* 15(3): 11–40.

24 Agamben, Giorgio (1998). *Homo Sacer: Sovereign Power and Bare Life*. Stanford: Stanford University Press.

25 Abujidi, Nurhan (2009). The Palestinian States of Exception and Agamben. *Contemporary Arab Affairs* 2(2): 272–91.

26 Shlaim, Avi (2000). *The Iron Wall: Israel and the Arab World*. London: Allen Lane, The Penguin Press.

27 Jeffris, D. C. (2012). The 'Center of Life Policy': Institutionalizing Statelessness in East Jerusalem. *Jerusalem Quarterly* 93: 94–103.

28 Raz, Avi (2012). *The Bride and the Dowry: Israel, Jordan and the Palestinians in the Aftermath of the June 1967 War*. New Haven: Yale University Press.

29 In the September 17 letter, Carter acknowledged:
- Arab Jerusalem is an integral part of the West Bank. Legal and historical Arab rights in the city must be respected and restored.
- Arab Jerusalem should be under Arab sovereignty.
- The Palestinian inhabitants of Arab Jerusalem are entitled to exercise their legitimate national rights, as part of the Palestinian People in the West Bank.
- Relevant Security Council resolutions related to Jerusalem, and Resolutions 242 and 267 in particular, must be applied. All measures taken by Israel to alter the status of the City are null and void and should be rescinded.

- All peoples must have free access to the City and enjoy the free exercises of worship and the right to visit and transit to the holy places without distinction or discrimination.
- The holy places of each faith may be placed under the administration and control of their representatives.
- Essential functions in the City should be undivided. A joint municipal council composed of an equal number of Arab and Israeli members can supervise the carrying out of these functions. This will enable the city to remain undivided.

30 Savir, Uri (1998). *The Process: 1,100 Days That Changed the Middle East.* New York: Random House.

31 Israel Ministry of Foreign Affairs (1996). Speech by PM-Elect Netanyahu-2 June. https://www.mfa.gov.il/mfa/mfa-archive/1996/pages /speech%20by%20pm-elect%20netanyahu%20-%20june%202-%201996 .aspx (accessed 19 June 2021).

32 Bishara, Marwan (2001). *Palestine/Israel: Peace or Apartheid: Prospects for Resolving the Conflict.* London: Zed Books.

33 OCHA (2008). Closure Update: Main Findings and Analysis, 30 April–11 September, Jerusalem, September 2008, 4–5.

34 Palestinian Center for Policy and Survey. Public Opinion Poll No (63), 14 March 2017.

35 Zureik, E. (2016). *Israel's Colonial Project in Palestine: Brutal Pursuit.* Abingdon: Routledge.

36 OCHA (2011). East Jerusalem: Key Humanitarian Concerns Special Focus, March. United Nations, OCHA. http://www.ochaopt.org/ documents/ocha_opt_jerusalem_report_2011_03_23_web_english.pdf.

37 Berda, Yael (2017). *Living Emergency: Israel's Permit Regime in the Occupied West Bank.* Stanford: Stanford University Press.

38 The Legal Center for Arab Minority Rights in Israel (ADALA) (2012). Family Reunification, 22 April. https://www.adalah.org/en/content/view /7556 (accessed 18 July 2020).

39 Savir, Uri (1998). *The Process: 1,100 Days That Changed the Middle East.* New York: Random House.

40 BBC News (2021). Palestinian Elections: Abbas Postpones Rare Polls, 29 April. https://www.bbc.co.uk/news/world-middle-east-56929547 (accessed 19 June 2021).

41 HaMoKed (2020). Center for the Defence of the Individual, 28. http://
    www.hamoked.org/Document.aspx?dID=Updates2174 (accessed 20 July
    2020).

42 Issued by HaMoked: Center for the Defence of the Individual, Adalah –
    The Legal Center for Arab Minority Rights in Israel, and Association for
    Civil Rights in Israel (ACRI).

43 HaMoKed (2018). Center for the Defence of the Individual, Press
    Release, 08 August. http://www.hamoked.org/Document.aspx?dID
    =Updates1961 (accessed 20 July 2020).

44 Al Jazeera (2021). Israeli Government Fails to Extend Controversial
    Citizenship Law, 06 July. https://www.aljazeera.com/news/2021/7/6/
    israeli-government-fails-to-extend-controversial-citizenship-law.

45 Center of the Defence of the Individuals (HaMoked) (2022). To the
    Minister of Interior, the Knesset and the Attorney General: Cancel the
    Amendment Allowing Revocation of Permanent Status of the Indigenous
    Palestinian Population of East Jerusalem, 13 September. https://hamoked
    .org/document.php?dID=Updates2331 (accessed 23 December 2022).

46 Al Jazeera (2019). PA condemns US Envoys' Presence at Israeli Settler-
    Linked Event, 30 June. https://www.aljazeera.com/news/middleeast
    /2019/06/pa-condemns-envoys-presence-israeli-settler-linked-event
    -190630152025683.html (accessed 18 June 2021).

47 Khalid, not his real name, Kufr 'Aqab resident, Jerusalem ID married to
    West Bank ID, WhatsApp conversation, 16 August 2021.

48 Hammoudeh, D., Hamayel, L. and Welchman, L. (2016). Beyond the
    Physicality of Space: East Jerusalem, Kufr 'Aqab, and the Politics of
    Everyday Suffering. *The Jerusalem Quarterly* 65: 35–60.

49 Tufajki, Khalil (2000). 'Settlements: A Geographic and Demographic
    Barrier to Peace. *Palestine-Israel Journal, of Political, Economics and
    Culture* 7(3 and 4): 52–8.

50 Alsaafin, Lenah (2021). What is Happening in Occupied East Jerusalem's
    Sheikh Jarrah? *Al Jazeera*, 01 May. https://www.aljazeera.com/news/2021
    /5/1/what-is-happening-in-occupied-east-jerusalems-sheikh-jarrah (20
    June 2021).

51 Ophir, A., Givoni, M. and Hanafl, S. (eds) (2009). *The Power of Inclusive
    Exclusion: Anatomy of Israeli Rule in the Occupied Palestinian Territories*.
    New York: Zone Books.

52 Ir Amim (n.d.). The Separation Barrier. https://www.ir-amim.org.il/en/ issue/separation-barrier (accessed 20 June 2021).

53 Salma, not her real name, housewife and resident of Kufr ʿAqab. She has a West Bank ID and her husband and children have Jerusalem IDs. WhatsApp conversation, 09 August 2021.

54 Farrell, Stephen, Lubell, Maayan and Auyyub, Rami (2020). Exclusive: Israel Builds New Jerusalem Road that will Link Settlements as Government Weighs West Bank Annexation. *Reuters*, 15 June. https:// www.reuters.com/article/us-israel-palestinians-road-exclusive -idUSKBN23M1LM (accessed 19 June 2021).

55 Munir Zughayer, an activist, chairperson of the local neighbourhood committees of north Jerusalem. WhatsApp conversation, 05 August 2021.

56 Association for Civil Rights in Israel (ACRI) (2017). Implications of Establishing a Separate Local Authority for the Neighborhoods Beyond the Barrier in Jerusalem. Position Paper, November. https://law.acri.org.il /en/wp-content/uploads/2017/11/Separate-Municiplaity-Position-Paper -1.pdf (19 June 2021).

57 Munir Zughayer, an activist, chairperson of the local neighbourhood committees of north Jerusalem. WhatsApp conversation, 05 August 2021.

58 Jamal Jumaʾ, coordinator of Palestinian Anti-Apartheid Wall grassroots campaign. Zoom interview, 15 August 2021.

59 Khalid, not his real name, Kufr ʿAqab resident, Jerusalem ID married to West Bank ID, WhatsApp conversation, 16 August 2021.

60 Munir Zughayer, an activist, chairperson of the local neighbourhood committees of north Jerusalem. WhatsApp conversation, 05 August 2021.

61 Magid, Jacob (2021). Israel Backs Off Housing Project at Jerusalem's Atarot Airport Site amid US Pressure. *The Times of Israel*, 25 November. https://www.timesofisrael.com/israel-backs-off-controversial-east -jerusalem-housing-project-amid-us-pressure/.

62 ARIJ (2012). Kafr ʿAqab Village Profile. Applied Research Institute Jerusalem.

63 Anonymous, pharmacist and researcher. Zoom interview, 03 August 2021.

64 Ola Awad-Shakhshir, minister of Palestinian Central Bureau of Statistics, Zoom interview, 16 December 2021.

65 Benvenisti, Meron (1995). *Intimate Enemies: Jews and Arabs in a Shared Land*. California: University of California Press.

66 Munir Zughayer, an activist, chairperson of the local neighbourhood committees of north Jerusalem. WhatsApp conversation, 05 August 2021.

67 Foucault, M. (2003). *Society must be Defended: Lectures at the Collège de France, 1975–76*. Picador.

68 Mbembe, A. (2003). Necropolitics. *Public Culture* 15(3): 11–40.

69 Abu Toumeh, Khaled (2021). Residents welcome PA policemen in Jerusalem Village. *The Jerusalem Post*, 06 January. https://www.jpost.com/israel-news/residents-welcome-pa-policemen-in-jerusalem-village-654136.

70 Jamal Juma', coordinator of Palestinian Anti-Apartheid Wall grassroots campaign. Zoom interview, 15 August 2021.

71 Khalid, not his real name, Kufr 'Aqab resident, Jerusalem ID married to West Bank ID, WhatsApp conversation, 16 August 2021.

72 Rula, not her real name, pharmacist and researcher. Zoom interview, 03 August 2021.

73 Mona, not her real name, housewife and resident of Kufr 'Aqab, she holds Jerusalem ID, her husband and children West Bank IDs, WhatsApp conversation, 06 August 2021.

74 B'Tselem (2017). East Jerusalem, 11 November. https://www.btselem.org/jerusalem (accessed 18 July 2020).

75 Rula, not her real name, pharmacist and researcher. Zoom interview, 03 August 2021.

76 Jamal Juma', coordinator of Palestinian Anti-Apartheid Wall grassroots campaign. Zoom interview, 15 August 2021.

77 Dajani, M., De Leo, D. and AlKhalidi, N. (2013). Planned Informality as a By-Product of the Occupation: The Case of Kufr Aqab Neighborhood in Jerusalem North. *Planum* 26(1): 1–10.

78 Munir Zughayer, an activist, chairperson of the local neighbourhood committees of north Jerusalem. WhatsApp conversation, 05 August 2021.

79 Al-Tamimi, Abd Al-Rahman (2021). Palestinian Water: From Control to Annexation (Arabic). Institute of Palestine Studies.

80 This is separate from a more general pattern in which the lack of services from the Jerusalem municipality cause residents to turn to the PA in order to obtain them. For example, after Bezeq, the Israeli communication network, stopped providing maintenance, residents turned to PA Telecom instead.

81 Amnesty International (2017). The Occupation of Water, 29 November. https://www.amnesty.org/en/latest/campaigns/2017/11/the-occupation -of-water/.

82 Ibrahim, not his real name, Kufr 'Aqab resident, West Bank ID married to Jerusalem ID, Messenger conversation, 10 August 2021.

83 Ibrahim, not his real name, Kufr 'Aqab resident, West Bank ID married to Jerusalem ID, Messenger conversation, 10 August 2021.

84 Selby, Jan (2005). The Political Economy of the Israeli-Palestinian Peace Process: An Introduction. Paper for Panel on the Political Economy of Conflict Transformation, International Studies Association, Hawaii, 1st–5th March, 1–24.

85 Tagari, Ehud and Oppenheimer, Yudith (2015). *Displaced in Their Own City: The Impact of Israeli policy in East Jerusalem on the Palestinian Neighborhoods of the City beyond the Separation Barrier.* Jerusalem: Ir Amin.

86 Mona, not her real name, housewife and resident of Kufr 'Aqab, she holds Jerusalem ID, her husband and children West Bank IDs, WhatsApp conversation, 06 August 2021.

87 Khalid, not his real name, Kufr 'Aqab resident, Jerusalem ID married to West Bank ID, WhatsApp conversation, 16 August 2021.

88 Ibrahim, not his real name, Kufr 'Aqab resident, West Bank ID married to Jerusalem ID, Messenger conversation, 10 August 2021.

89 Khalid, not his real name, Kufr 'Aqab resident, Jerusalem ID married to West Bank ID, WhatsApp conversation, 16 August 2021.

90 Ashly, Jaclynn (2018). Palestinians in Kufr 'Aqab: 'We live here just to wait'. *Aljazeera*, 07 January. https://www.aljazeera.com/news/2018/1/7/palestinians -in-kufr-aqab-we-live-here-just-to-wait (accessed 18 June 2021).

91 Rula, not her real name, pharmacist and researcher. Zoom interview, 03 August 2021.

92 This use of uncertainty is a key part of Israel's strategy and extends to its negotiating position/s – for example, the chief Israeli negotiator Uri

Savir once told Ahmed Qurei, his Palestinian counterpart, that 'even if we negotiated for a thousand year, Israel will not reveal the map for the final stage of redeployment' (2005: 348). See Quray', Aḥmad (2005). *al-Riwāyah al-Filasṭīnīyah al-kāmilah lil-mufāwaḍāt: min Ūslū ilá Kharīṭat al-ṭarīq.* Vol. 1. Bayrūt: Mu'assasat al-Dirāsāt al-Filasṭīnīyah.

93   Abu Hatoum, N. (2021). For 'a no-state yet to come': Palestinian Urban Place-Making in Kufr Aqab, Jerusalem. *Environment and Planning E: Nature and Space* 4(1): 85–108.

94   Rula, not her real name, pharmacist and researcher. Zoom interview, 03 August 2021.

95   Hamayel, L., Hammoudeh, D. and Welchman, L. (2017). Reproductive Health and Rights in East Jerusalem: The Effects of Militarisation and Biopolitics on the Experiences of Pregnancy and Birth of Palestinians Living in the Kufr 'Aqab neighbourhood. *Reproductive Health Matters* 25(sup1): 87–95.

96   Berda, Yael (2017). *Living Emergency: Israel's Permit Regime in the Occupied West Bank.* Redwood City: Stanford University Press.

97   Weizman, Eyal (2007). *Hollow Land: Israel's Architecture of Occupation.* London: Verso Books. Halper, J. (2015). *War Against the People: Israel, the Palestinians and Global Pacification.* London: Pluto Press.

98   Foucault, M. (1991). *Discipline and Punish: The Birth of a Prison.* London: Penguin.

99   Khalid, not his real name, Kufr 'Aqab resident, Jerusalem ID married to West Bank ID, WhatsApp conversation, 16 August 2021.

100 Society of St. Yves is a Catholic human rights organization. Another great legal achievement for St Yves in the field of Health insurance for people with family unification, 21 September 2021. https://www.saintyves.org/news/another-great-legal-achievement-for-st-yves-in-the-field-of-health-insurance-for-people-with-family-unification.html.

101 Amnesty International (2022). Israel's Apartheid Against Palestinians: Cruel System of Domination and Crime against Humanity, February. https://www.amnesty.org/en/latest/campaigns/2022/02/israels-system-of-apartheid/.

102 Hamayel, L., Hammoudeh, D. and Welchman, L. (2017). Reproductive Health and Rights in East Jerusalem: The Effects of Militarisation and Biopolitics on the Experiences of Pregnancy and Birth of Palestinians

Living in the Kufr 'Aqab Neighbourhood. *Reproductive Health Matters* 25(sup1): 87–95.

103 WAFA News Agency (2021). Israel Punitively Revokes Health Insurance of 16 Former Prisoners from Jerusalem, 27 May. https://english.wafa.ps/Pages/Details/124769.

104 Hammoudeh, D., Hamayel, L. and Welchman, L. (2016). Beyond the Physicality of Space: East Jerusalem, Kufr 'Aqab, and the Politics of Everyday Suffering. *The Jerusalem Quarterly* 65: 35–60.

105 Khalid, not his real name, Kufr 'Aqab resident, Jerusalem ID married to West Bank ID, WhatsApp conversation, 16 August 2021.

106 Alzajeera (2021). In Pictures: In Show of Unity, Palestinians go on Strike, 18 May. https://www.aljazeera.com/gallery/2021/5/18/in-pictures-palestinians-unite-with-a-general-strike.

107 Rula, not her real name, pharmacist and researcher. Zoom interview, 03 August 2021.

108 Mona, not her real name, housewife and resident of Kufr 'Aqab, she holds Jerusalem ID, her husband and children West Bank IDs, WhatsApp conversation, 06 August 2021.

109 Rula, not her real name, pharmacist and researcher. Zoom interview, 03 August 2021.

110 Rula, not her real name, pharmacist and researcher. Zoom interview, 03 August 2021.

111 Independent (2021). Israel Rebuffs WHO Vaccine Request for Palestinian Medics, Amid Outcry over Disparity, 08 January. https://www.independent.co.uk/news/world/middle-east/israel-palestine-coronavirus-vaccine-b1784474.html?fbclid=IwAR2Sut7ykl7PAw1W4y66sBjedlhRtWgfkeWjLPqkMDs-sbXBWkoPmUxnbMQ.

112 Independent (2021). Israel Rebuffs WHO Vaccine Request for Palestinian Medics, Amid Outcry over Disparity, 08 January. https://www.independent.co.uk/news/world/middle-east/israel-palestine-coronavirus-vaccine-b1784474.html?fbclid=IwAR2Sut7ykl7PAw1W4y66sBjedlhRtWgfkeWjLPqkMDs-sbXBWkoPmUxnbMQ.

113 Jewish News (2021). Yuli Edelstein: It's in Our Interest Not Our Obligation to Get Palestinians Jabs, 24 January. https://jewishnews.timesofisrael.com/yuli-edelstein-its-our-interest-not-our-obligation-to-give-palestinians-jabs/.

114 Salma, not her real name, housewife and resident of Kufr 'Aqab. She
has West Bank ID and her husband and children have Jerusalem ID
WhatsApp conversation, 09 August 2021.

115 Ynet News. Lukash, Alexandra and Yanko, Adir (2020). Gamzu Slams
Arab Community for 'coronavirus terrorism'. Ynet News, 16 August.
https://www.ynetnews.com/article/BJkbWP8Mw.

116 Uddin, Rayhan and Osman, Nadda (2021). Palestinians in Jerusalem
'not afraid' of Threatening Texts from 'Israeli intelligence'. Middle East
Eye, 11 May. https://www.middleeasteye.net/news/israel-jerusalem
-intelligence-threat-text-message-palestine-aqsa (accessed 22 June 2021).

117 Shalhoub-Kevorkian, N. (2015). *Security Theology, Surveillance and
the Politics of Fear*. Cambridge Studies in Law and Society. Cambridge:
Cambridge University Press.

118 Shalhoub-Kevorkian, N. (2015). *Security Theology, Surveillance and
the Politics of Fear*. Cambridge Studies in Law and Society. Cambridge:
Cambridge University Press.

119 Hasson, Nir (2020). Israel Shuts Palestinian Coronavirus Testing Clinic
in East Jerusalem. *Haaretz*, 15 April. https://www.haaretz.com/israel
-news/.premium-israeli-police-raid-palestinian-coronavirus-testing
-clinic-in-east-jerusalem-1.8767788.

120 The Legal Center for Arab Minority Rights in Israel (Adalah) (2020).
Adalah files urgent Israeli Supreme Court petition: Coronavirus testing
for 150,000 Palestinians in East Jerusalem, 08 April. https://www.adalah
.org/en/content/view/9975 (accessed 20 July 2020).

121 Munir Zughayer, an activist, chairperson of the local neighbourhood
committees of north Jerusalem. WhatsApp conversation, 05 August 2021.

122 Adalah (2020). The Legal Center for Arab Minority Rights in Israel.
Following Adalah's Supreme Court Petition, Israel to Open Coronavirus
Testing Centers in East Jerusalem Neighborhoods beyond the Separation
Wall, 14 April. https://www.adalah.org/en/content/view/9979.

123 Adalah (2020). The Legal Center for Arab Minority Rights in Israel.
Following Adalah's Supreme Court Petition, Israel to Open Coronavirus
Testing Centers in East Jerusalem Neighborhoods beyond the Separation
Wall, 14 April. https://www.adalah.org/en/content/view/9979.

124 Adalah (2021). The Legal Center for Arab Minority Rights in Israel.
Adalah Demands Israel Provide Immediate COVID-19 Vaccines for

Palestinian Jerusalemites Living behind Separation Wall, 14 January. https://www.adalah.org/en/content/view/10224.

125 Rula, not her real name, pharmacist and researcher. Zoom interview, 03 August 2021.

126 Ferwana, Abdelnasser (2021). COVID-19 Tightens Its Grip on Prisoners and Exacerbates Their Suffering. Institute for Palestine Studies, 04 February. https://www.palestine-studies.org/en/node/1650969.

127 Boxerman, Aaron (2021). With Distrust Rampant, East Jerusalem Palestinians Shirk COVID Vaccine. *The Times of Israel*, 06 January. https://www.timesofisrael.com/with-distrust-rampant-east-jerusalem -palestinians-shirk-covid-vaccine/.

128 Munir Zughayer, an activist, chairperson of the local neighbourhood committees of north Jerusalem. WhatsApp conversation, 05 August 2021.

129 Mona, not her real name, Kufr 'Aqab resident, West Bank ID married to Jerusalem ID, Messenger conversation, 06 August 2021.

130 Hashmonai, Adi (2021). Israeli City Barring Unvaccinated from Entry Accused of anti-Palestinian Discrimination, 06 August. https://www .haaretz.com/israel-news/.premium-acre-accused-of-anti-palestinian -discrimination-over-ban-on-entry-of-unvaccinated-1.10091624?fbclid =IwAR1imj2o-kBDSn63MLrYyg3y6UWWWRJHgFjMSwJV35q4bZqM pAifL7rcKf4.

131 United Nations, Department of Economic and Social Affairs (2020). The Impact of COVID-19 on Indigenous Peoples Policy Briefs, No. 70, 21 May. https://www.un.org/development/desa/dpad/wp-content/ uploads/sites/45/publication/PB_70.pdf.

132 Rula, not her real name, pharmacist and researcher. Zoom interview, 03 August 2021.

133 Jamal Juma', coordinator of Palestinian Anti-Apartheid Wall grassroots campaign. Zoom interview, 15 August 2021.

134 Jamal Juma', coordinator of Palestinian Anti-Apartheid Wall grassroots campaign. Zoom interview, 15 August 2021.

135 Rula, not her real name, pharmacist and researcher. Zoom interview, 03 August 2021.

136 Ibrahim, not his real name, Kufr 'Aqab resident, West Bank ID married to Jerusalem ID, Messenger conversation, 10 August 2021.

137 Rula, not her real name, pharmacist and researcher. Zoom interview, 03 August 2021.

138 Adalah (2020). The Legal Center for Arab Minority Rights in Israel. Report by Adalah to UN Special Rapporteurs and Independent Experts in response to Joint Questionnaire on COVID-19 and Human rights, 4 July. https://worldjusticeproject.org/sites/default/files/documents /Adalah%20UN%20COVID-19%20Report%20with%20Major %20Findings%2016.07.pdf.

139 Wade, Lizzie (2020). American Association for Advancement of Science (AAAS). COVID-19 Data on Native Americans is 'a National Disgrace.' This Scientist is Fighting to be Counted, 24 September. https://www .sciencemag.org/news/2020/09/covid-19-data-native-americans-national -disgrace-scientist-fighting-be-counted.

140 Ola Awad-Shakhshir, minister of Palestinian Central Bureau of Statistics, Zoom interview, 16 December 2021.

141 Greenberg, Joel (1997). Palestinian Census Ignites Controversy over Jerusalem. *The New York Times*, 11 December. https://www.nytimes .com/1997/12/11/world/palestinian-census-ignites-controversy-over -jerusalem.html.

142 Palestinian Central Bureau of Statistics (2020). A Tale of the Statistical Number. Ramallah - Palestine.

143 Husseini, Ibrahim. Israel Arrests Palestinians over Population Count. *Al-Jazeera*, 22 November 2017. https://www.aljazeera.com/news/2017/11 /22/israel-arrests-palestinians-over-population-count.

144 Palestinian Central Bureau of Statistics (2021). Jerusalem Statistical Yearbook 2021, No. 23. Ramallah – Palestine.

145 Mallard, A., Pesantes, M. A., Zavaleta-Cortijo, C. and Ward, J. (2021). An Urgent Call to Collect Data Related to COVID-19 and Indigenous Populations Globally. *BMJ Global Health* 6(3): e004655.

146 United Nations, Department of Economic and Social Affairs (2020). The Impact of COVID-19 on Indigenous Peoples Policy Briefs, No. 70, 21 May. https://www.un.org/development/desa/dpad/wp-content/ uploads/sites/45/publication/PB_70.pdf.

147 Alfred, Taiaiake (2005). *Wasáse: Indigenous Pathways of Action and Freedom.* Peterborough: Broadview Press.

148 Munir Zughayer, an activist, chairperson of the local neighbourhood committees of north Jerusalem. WhatsApp conversation, 05 August 2021.

149 Naser-Najjab, N. (2020). Palestinian Leadership and the Contemporary Significance of the First Intifada. *Race & Class* 62(2): 61–79.

150 Yiftachel, Oren (2009). Creeping Apartheid in Israel-Palestine. *Middle East Report* 253: 7–15. Benvenisti, Meron (2010). United We Stand: Do Israelis and Palestinians belong to One Divided Society, or to Two Separate Societies in a Situation of Forced Proximity as a Result of a Temporary Occupation? *Ha'aretz*, 28 January. Hilal, J. (2015). Rethinking Palestine: Settler-Colonialism, Neo-Liberalism and Individualism in the West Bank and Gaza Strip. *Contemporary Arab Affairs* 8(3): 351–62.

Chapter 5

1 Farrell, Stephen and Sawafta, Ali (2018). 'Prince William Pays First Official British Royal Visit to Occupied West Bank'. *Reuters*, 27 June. https://uk.reuters.com/article/uk-britain-royals-israel-palestinians/prince-william-pays-first-official-british-royal-visit-to-occupied-west-bank-idUKKBN1JN1B5 (accessed 18 July 2020).

2 Tanous, Izzat (1982). *ālflsṭynywn māḍ mǧyd wmstqbl bāhr*. Beirut: Research Center, Palestine Liberation Organization.

3 United Nations Relief and Works Agency for Palestine Refugees in the Near East (UNRWA). Who We Are. https://www.unrwa.org/who-we-are (accessed 15 July 2020).

4 Zureik, E. (2001). Constructing Palestine through Surveillance Practices. *British Journal of Middle Eastern Studies* 28(2): 205–27.

5 Abu Tair, Maher (2021). māḍā y'ny sqwṭ ālwkālﻪ? (What Does the Fall of UNRWA Mean?) Arabic. Al Maqar, 04 December. https://maqar.com/archives/512656.

6 Cook, Jonathan (2018). Is Leaked Document Trump's 'deal of the century?' *Middle East Eye*, 9 May. https://www.jonathan-cook.net/2019-05-09/is-leaked-document-trumps-deal-of-the-century/ (accessed 04 May 2020).

7 Beaumont, Peter and Holmes, Oliver (2018). US Confirms End to Funding for UN Palestinian Refugees. *The Guardian*, 31 August. https://www.theguardian.com/world/2018/aug/31/trump-to-cut-all-us-funding-for-uns-main-palestinian-refugee-programme (accessed 24 May 2019).

8 United Nations Relief and Works Agency for Palestine Refugees in the Near East (UNRWA) (2021). United States Announces Restoration

of U.S. $150 Million to Support Palestine Refugees, 07 April. https://
www.unrwa.org/newsroom/press-releases/united-states-announces
-restoration-us-150-million-support-palestine (accessed 04 September
2021).

9 Philippe Lazzarini, the agency's commissioner-general, welcomed this
decision, and said: 'UNRWA could not be more pleased that once again
we will partner with the United States to provide critical assistance to
some of the most vulnerable refugees across the Middle East and fulfil
our mandate to educate and provide primary health care to millions of
refugees every day.'

10 The Guardian (2021). UN Palestine Refugee Aid Agency 'Close to
Collapse' after Funding Cuts, 5 November. https://www.theguardian.com
/world/2021/nov/05/un-palestine-aid-agency-is-close-to-collapse-after
-funding-cuts (accessed 25 March 2022).

11 United Nations Relief and Works Agency for Palestine Refugees
(UNRWA) (2022). Message from UNRWA Commissioner-General to
Palestine Refugees, 23 April. https://www.unrwa.org/newsroom/official
-statements/message-unrwa-commissioner-general-palestine-refugees
(accessed 24 June 2022). The PLO claimed this proposal put UNRWA at
risk of being dissolved and urged the commissioner-general to withdraw
it – see I24News. Palestinians fear UNRWA taking steps to dissolve,
25 April 2022. https://www.i24news.tv/en/news/middle-east/palestinian
-territories/1650899570-palestinians-fear-unrwa-taking-steps-to-end
-services (accessed 09 September 2022).

12 Peace to Prosperity Plan (January 2020). Peace-to-Prosperity-0120.pdf
(archives.gov) (accessed 07 June 2021). The Peace to Prosperity Plan also
proposed the Jewish refugee 'problem' should be 'compartmentalized'
when it suggested it should be addressed through 'an appropriate
international mechanism separate from the Israel-Palestinian Peace
Agreement' (2020: 9).

13 Al Husseini, Jalal (2010). UNRWA and the Refugees: A Difficult but
Lasting Marriage. *Journal of Palestine Studies* 40: 1.

14 Sharett observed Jews who lived in other Arab countries were only
forced to leave after Israel was established. This, Shohat notes, 'brought
a painful binarism into the formerly peaceful relationship between the
two communities' (1988: 11). This, however, falls beyond the scope of

the current book. For a more thorough discussion, see Shiblak (1986); Massad (1996); Shohat (1988); and Naser-Najjab (2015). Also see Shohat, E. (1988). Sephardim in Israel: Zionism from the Standpoint of Its Jewish Victims. *Social Text* 19(20): 1–35.

15 Shenhav, Y. (1999). The Jews of Iraq, Zionist Ideology, and the Property of the Palestinian Refugees of 1948: An Anomaly of National Accounting. *International Journal of Middle East Studies* 31(4): 605–30.

16 And, of course, the use of the word 'problem' is entirely deserving of critical scrutiny and interrogation.

17 Khalidi, Rashid (2013). *Brokers of Deceit: How the US Has Undermined Peace in the Middle East.* Boston: Beacon Press.

18 Sayigh, R. (2008). *The Palestinians: From Peasants to Revolutionaries.* London: Bloomsbury Publishing.

19 Khalidi, Rashid I. (1992). Observations on the Right of Return. *Journal of Palestine Studies* 21, no. 2 (Winter): 29.

20 Masalha, Nur (2002). The Palestinian Nakba: Zionism, 'Transfer' and the 1948 Exodus, *Global Dialogue* 4 (Summer): 3; ProQuest Business Collection pg. 77.

21 Adalah (2020). The Legal Center for Arab Minority Rights. Israel's Jewish Nation-State Law, 20 December. https://www.adalah.org/en/content/view/9569 (accessed 23 February 2021).

22 Wootliff, Raoul (2019). The Times of Israel. Defending Nation-State Law, PM Says Israeli Arabs have 22 Other Countries, 11 March. https://www.timesofisrael.com/defending-nation-state-law-pm-says-israeli-arabs-have-22-other-countries/ (accessed 14 March 2021).

23 United Nations Relief and Works Agency for Palestine Refugees in the Near East (UNRWA) (2020). UNRWA COVID-19 appeal, August–December. https://www.unrwa.org/sites/default/files/content/resources/unrwa_covid-19_appeal_august-_december_2020.pdf (accessed 14 March 2021).

24 Human Rights Watch (2021). Lebanon: Refugees, Migrants Left Behind in Vaccine Rollout, 06 April. https://www.hrw.org/news/2021/04/06/lebanon-refugees-migrants-left-behind-vaccine-rollout (accessed 19 September 2021).

25 Reuters (2021). Palestinian Refugees in Lebanon Three Times more Likely to Die with COVID-19, 16 February. https://www.reuters.com/

article/us-lebanon-refugees-health-trfn-idUSKBN2AG22M (accessed 14 September 2021).

26 Aaraj, E., Haddad, P., Khalife, S., Fawaz, M. and Van Hout, M. C. (2021). Understanding and Responding to Substance Use and Abuse in the Palestinian Refugee Camps in Lebanon Prior to and During COVID-19 Times. *International Journal of Mental Health and Addiction*, 29: 1–17.

27 The United Nations Relief and Works Agency for Palestine Refugees (UNRWA) (n.d.). Jalazone Camp. https://www.unrwa.org/where-we-work/west-bank/jalazone-camp#block-menu-block-10 (accessed 14 March 2022).

28 The United Nations Relief and Works Agency for Palestine Refugees (UNRWA) (2021). A Day in the Life of a Palestine Refugee Student in the West Bank, 30 April. https://www.unrwa.org/newsroom/features/day-life-palestine-refugee-student-west-bank (accessed 14 September 2021).

29 Mbembe, A. (2003). Necropolitics. *Public Culture* 15(3): 11–40.

30 Mbembe, A. (2003). Necropolitics. *Public Culture* 15(3): 11–40.

31 Agamben, Giorgio (1998). *Homo Sacer: Sovereign Power and Bare Life*. Stanford: Stanford University Press.

32 Dina, not her real name, nurse, Jalazone, Zoom interview, 15 December 2021.

33 Layla, not her real name, kindergarten teacher, Jalazone, Zoom Interview, 03 January 2022.

34 Ahmad Dalashi, internal medicine doctor, Ramallah Hospital and the Medical chief of the coronavirus emergency committee in Jalazone Camp. Zoom interview, 30 January 2022.

35 B'Tselem (2018). The Israeli Information Center for Human Rights in the Occupied Territories. Life under Shadow of Beit El Settlement: Travel Restrictions on Residents of al-Jalazun R.C., 13 March. https://www.btselem.org/freedom_of_movement/20180313_jalazun_travel_restrictions (accessed 14 September 2021).

36 Mbembe, A. (2003). Necropolitics. *Public Culture* 15(3): 11–40.

37 Agamben, G. (1998). *Homo Sacer: Sovereign Power and Bare Life*. Stanford: Stanford University Press.

38 Agamben, G. (1998). *Homo Sacer: Sovereign Power and Bare Life*. Stanford: Stanford University Press.

39 Shalhoub-Kevorkian, N. (2015). *Security Theology, Surveillance and the Politics of Fear*. Cambridge Studies in Law and Society. Cambridge: Cambridge University Press.

40 Fanon, Franz (1963). *The Wretched of the Earth*. New York: Grove Press.

41 Foucault, M. (1995). *Discipline and Punish: The Birth of the Prison*. New York: Vintage Books.

42 Hanafi, Sari (2009). Spacio-Cide: Colonial Politics, Invisibility and Rezoning in Palestinian Territory. *Contemporary Arab Affairs* 2(1): 106–21.

43 Agamben, G. (1995). We Refugees. Translated by Michael Rocke. *Symposium* 49(2): 114–19. http://www.egs.edu/faculty/agamben/agamben-we-refugees.html (accessed 14 September 2021).

44 Sayigh, R. (2008). *The Palestinians: From Peasants to Revolutionaries*. London: Bloomsbury Publishing.

45 Haddad, Toufic (2016). *Palestine Ltd: Neoliberalism and Nationalism in the Occupied Territories* London: I. B. Taurus.

46 Badarin, Emile (2015). Settler-Colonialist Management of Entrances to the Native Urban Space in Palestine. *Settler Colonial Studies* 5(3): 226–35.

47 Hilal, Jamil (2015). Rethinking Palestine: Settler-Colonialism, Neoliberalism and Individualism in the West Bank and Gaza Strip. *Contemporary Arab Affairs* 8(3): 1–12. (accessed 17 November 2021). doi: 10.1080/17550912.2015.1052226. Turner, Mandy (2012). Completing the Circle: Peacebuilding as Colonial Practice in the Occupied Palestinian Territory. *International Peacekeeping* 19(4): 492–507. DOI: 10.1080/13533312.2012.709774.

48 Haddad, Toufic (2016). *Palestine Ltd: Neoliberalism and Nationalism in the Occupied Territories*. London: I. B. Taurus.

49 Karim, not his real name, resident of Jalazone, 05 September 2020. Telephone conversation.

50 Karim, not his real name, resident of Jalazone, 05 January 2020. Telephone conversation.

51 And not without good reason. Although Arab leaders frequently sought to co-opt the Palestinian 'cause' for their own purposes, their interests often diverged, as the events of Black September clearly illustrated. Hilal demonstrates this by referring to the changes that Jordan made in the West Bank after it took control of this territory in 1948. He observes: '[U]nder Jordanian rule, elites kept the family dimension, MPs, ministerial positions [and] renewed [the] influence of traditional families in the WB. On the other hand, Jordanian rule weakened the influence of

Jerusalemite families in Jerusalem and the role of religious organizations (2002: 31)'.

52 Al Najjar, Shadi. A Member of Board of Directors, Jalazone Volunteer Work Youth. Zoom interview, 07 January 2021.

53 Hanafi, S., Chaaban, J. and Seyfert, K. (2012). Social Exclusion of Palestinian Refugees in Lebanon: Reflections on the Mechanisms that Cement their Persistent Poverty. *Refugee Survey Quarterly* 31(1): 34–53.

54 The United Nations Relief and Works Agency for Palestine Refugees (UNRWA). A Day in the Life of a Palestine Refugee Student in the West Bank, 30 April 2021. https://www.unrwa.org/newsroom/features/day-life -palestine-refugee-student-west-bank.

55 Shadi Al Najjar, a member of Board of Directors, Jalazone Volunteer Work Youth. Zoom interview, 07 January 2021.

56 Nofel, Aziz (2020). West Bank Camps, Disappointed with UNRWA, Take Initiative to Fight Coronavirus. Al Monitor, 27 March. https://www .al-monitor.com/originals/2020/03/palestinian-refugee-camps-unrwa -measures-coronavirus.html (08 September 2020).

57 Al Husseini, Jalal (2010). UNRWA and the Refugees: A Difficult but Lasting Marriage. *Journal of Palestine Studies* 40: 1. Irfan, A. (2018). Internationalising Palestine: UNRWA and Palestinian Nationalism in the Refugee Camps, 1967-82 (Doctoral dissertation, The London School of Economics and Political Science (LSE)).

58 Al Husseini, Jalal (2010). UNRWA and the Refugees: A Difficult but Lasting Marriage. *Journal of Palestine Studies* 40: 1.

59 Shadi Al Najjar. Zoom interview, 07 January 2021.

60 A member of Jalazone Volunteer Work Youth.

61 Moussa Qattash, a member of Jalazone Volunteer Work Youth. Zoom interview, 07 January 2021.

62 United Nations Office for the Coordination of Humanitarian Affairs (OCHA) (2020b). Unprotected: Settler Attacks against Palestinians on the Rise Amidst the Outbreak of COVID-19, 22 June. https://www .ochaopt.org/content/unprotected-settler-attacks-against-palestinians -rise-amidst-outbreak-covid-19 (accessed June 2020).

63 Moussa Qattash, a member of Jalazone Volunteer Work Youth. Zoom interview, 07 January 2021.

64 Ramallah News (2020). The Minister of Health Instructs to Provide
    the Needs of Al-Jalazone to Confront Corona (Arabic), 11 July. https://
    ramallah.news/post/ (06 September 2020).

65 Some donors responded to the allegation that Palestinian textbooks incite
    hatred against Israel by reallocating funding– see Naser-Najjab, N. and
    Pappé, I. (2016). Palestine: Reframing Palestine in the Post-Oslo period.
    In Robert Guyver (ed.) *Teaching History and the Changing Nation State:
    Transnational and Intranational Perspectives*. Bloomsbury Academic.

66 United Nation (2021), General Assembly. Human Rights Council.
    Forty-sixth session 22 February–19 March 2021. Written Statement
    Submitted by United Nations Watch, a Non-governmental Organization
    in Special Consultative Status, 01 February. https://www.un.org/unispal
    /wp-content/uploads/2021/03/AHRC46NGO136_170321.pdf (accessed
    09 November 2021).

67 The United Nations Relief and Works Agency for Palestine Refugees
    (UNRWA) (2021). UNRWA Statement on the latest European Parliament
    Resolution, Official Statements, 30 April. https://www.unrwa.org
    /newsroom/official-statements/unrwa-statement-latest-european
    -parliament-resolution.

68 Harkov, Lahav (2021). EU Finally Releases Report of Incitement,
    Antisemitism in PA Textbooks, June. *The Jerusalem Post* 20. https://
    www.jpost.com/diaspora/antisemitism/eu-releases-report-of-incitement
    -antisemitism-in-palestinian-textbooks-671534 (accessed 09 November
    2021).

69 Medical Aid for Palestinians (MAP) (2021). MAP Calls on UK
    Government to Reverse Aid Cuts to Palestinian Healthcare,
    18 November. https://www.map.org.uk/news/archive/post/1309-map
    -calls-on-uk-government-to-reverse-aid-cuts-to-palestinian-healthcare
    (accessed 06 February 2022).

70 Abed Elrazik, Adnan, Amin, Riyad and Davis, Uri (1978). Problems of
    Palestinians in Israel, Land, Work, Education. *Journal of Palestine Studies*
    7, no. 3 (spring): 31–54.

71 Bashour, Najla, (1971). The Alteration of the School Curricula in the
    West Bank of Jordan after 1967 [in Arabic]. Shu'un Filastiniyyah 3
    (1971): 229–41.

72 Piterberg, Gabriel (2008). *The Returns of Zionism: Myths, Politics
    and Scholarship in Israel*. London: Verso. Bashour, Najla (1971). The

Alteration of the School Curricula in the West Bank of Jordan after 1967 [in Arabic]. *Shu'un Filastiniyyah* 3 (1971): 229–41.

73 Ahmad Dalashi, internal medicine doctor, Ramallah Hospital and the medical chief of the coronavirus emergency committee in Jalazone Camp. Zoom interview, 30 January 2022.

74 World Health Organization. Coronavirus Disease (COVID-19) Advice for the Public. https://www.who.int/emergencies/diseases/novel -coronavirus-2019/advice-for-public (accessed 15 July 2020).

75 Ahmad Dalashi, internal medicine doctor, Ramallah Hospital and the medical chief of the coronavirus emergency committee in Jalazone Camp. Zoom interview, 30 January 2022.

76 Al Khatib, I. and Tabakhna, H. (2006). Housing Conditions and Health in Jalazone Refugee Camp in Palestine. *East Mediterranean Health Journal* 12: 144–52.

77 Hilal, Jamil (ed.) (2020). *Isolation, Separation and Quarantine*. Palestine: Qattan Foundation.

78 Ahmad Dalashi, internal medicine doctor, Ramallah Hospital and the medical chief of the coronavirus emergency committee in Jalazone Camp. Zoom interview, 30 January 2022.

79 Middle East Monitor (2020). Palestinian Refugee Camps in Lebanon Are Facing Covid-19 Alone, 14 October. https://www.middleeastmonitor .com/20201014-palestinian-refugee-camps-in-lebanon-are-facing-covid -19-alone/ (accessed 30 May 2021).

80 Samah, not her name, kindergarten teacher, Jalazone, Zoom interview, 03 January 2022.

81 Dina, not her real name, nurse, Jalazone, Zoom interview, 15 December 2021.

82 Al Najjar, interview.

83 Florey, Katherine (2022). The Tribal COVID-19 Response. *Regulatory Review*, 17 March. https://www.theregreview.org/2021/03/17/florey -tribal-covid-19-response/ (accessed 15 August 2022).

84 In 1996, the PLO reactivated the Refugee Affairs Department and formed popular committees who helped to improve camp services.

85 Refugee Affairs Department (2018). PLO, Goals, Initiatives and Program, 19 September. http://plord.ps/post/7692/

86 The hospital is located in Turmus 'Ayya village. The project began in 2016 with the support of the Venezuelan government (who allocated

$15 million) and Palestinians from Turmus 'Ayya (who donated land). The Palestinian Economic Council for Development and Reconstruction (PECDAR). The Hugo Chavez Ophthalmic Hospital. http://www.pecdar .ps/en/article/926/The-Hugo-Chavez-Ophthalmic-Hospital- (accessed 15 August 2022).

87 Ahmad Dalashi, internal medicine doctor, Ramallah Hospital and the medical chief of the coronavirus emergency committee in Jalazone Camp. Zoom interview, 30 January 2022.

88 Naser-Najjab, N. (2020). Palestinian Leadership and the Contemporary Significance of the First Intifada. *Race & Class* 62(2): 61–79.

89 Dr Abdelrahman Tamimi, assistant professor of strategic planning and future studies at the Arab American University. An expert in the field of water resources. Zoom interview, 27 April 2022.

90 FACTS Information Committee (1988). 'Towards a State of Independence: The Palestinian Uprising, December 1987–August 1988' Jerusalem. http://www.jmcc.org/Documentsandmaps.aspx?id=609.

91 Dina, not her real name, nurse, Jalazone, Zoom interview, 15 December 2021.

92 Karim, resident of Jalazone, Telephone conversation 05 September 2020.

93 Ahmad Dalashi, internal medicine doctor, Ramallah Hospital and the medical chief of the coronavirus emergency committee in Jalazone Camp. Zoom interview, 30 January 2022.

94 Shadi Al Najjar, a member of Board of Directors, Jalazone Volunteer Work Youth. Zoom interview, 07 January 2021.

95 Tabner, Isaac T. (2020). Five Ways Coronavirus Lockdowns Increase Inequality. *The Conversation*, 8 April. https://theconversation.com/five -ways-coronavirus-lockdowns-increase-inequality-135767 (accessed 15 August 2022).

96 Sharif, Maher (2020). How Will the World After Corona Be?, Institute of Palestine Studies blog, 22 May (Arabic).

97 Jalazone was established on 253 dunums of land in 1948. Samah, kindergarten teacher, Jalazone, Zoom Interview, 03 January 2022. The United Nations Relief and Works Agency for Palestine Refugees (UNRWA) (2005). The Jalazone Refugee Camp, 31 March. https://web .archive.org/web/20070310131014/http:/www.un.org:80/unrwa/refugees/ westbank/jalazone.html (accessed 12 April 2021).

98 Ahmad Dalashi, internal medicine doctor, Ramallah Hospital and the medical chief of the coronavirus emergency committee in Jalazone Camp. Zoom interview, 30 January 2022.

99 Shadi Al Najjar, a member of board of directors, Jalazone Volunteer Work Youth. Zoom interview, 07 January 2021.

100 Dr Abdelrahman Tamimi, assistant professor of strategic planning and future studies at the Arab American University. An expert in the field of water resources. Zoom interview, 27 April 2022.

101 Palestinian Environmental NGOs Network (PENGON) (2018). Wastewater Flow from 'Merav' & 'Ma'ali Jalbua', Settlements Turn Jalboun Village to Epidemic Area, 31 January. http://www.pengon.org/articles/view/42 (accessed 12 April 2021).

102 Wafi, Ali and Ziadeh, Saad eddin (2020). The Necessity for Food Sovereignty in Gaza in the Light of the Corona Pandemic. Palestinian Environmental NGOs Network (PENGON). http://www.pengon.org/uploads/Food%20Sovereignty.pdf (accessed 15 August 2022).

103 Human Rights Watch (2021). A Threshold Crossed, Israeli Authorities and the Crimes of Apartheid and Persecution. israel_palestine0421_reportcover_8.5x11 (hrw.org). (accessed 15 August 2022) Abu-Sada, C. (2009). Cultivating Dependence: Palestinian Agriculture under the Israeli Occupation. In Ophir, A., Givoni, M. and Hanafi, S. (eds), *The Power of Inclusive Exclusion: Anatomy of Israeli Rule in the Occupied Palestinian Territories*. New York: Zone Books, 413–34.

104 PENGON- FoE Palestine was established in 1996 to promote environmental sustainability by coordinating the work of Palestinian NGOs who work in this area. The network emerged after a number of NGOs stressed there was '[an] urgent need to protect our environment and face [e]nvironmental violations'. http://www.pengon.org/articles/view/1.

105 The Jerusalem water undertaking was founded in 1949. Israel took control of it in 1967. https://www.jwu.org/jwu/?p=1698&lang=en.

106 A B'Tselem report (2009) observes that while Israel views facilities built in the West Bank as part of its local waste management system, 'it applies less rigorous regulatory standards there than it does inside its own territory – see 'B'Tselem – The Israeli Information Center for Human Rights in the Occupied Territories. Made in Israel: Exploiting Palestinian

Land for Treatment of Israeli Waste, December 2017. 'B'Tselem (2018). The Israeli Information Center for Human Rights in the Occupied Territories. Made in Israel: Exploiting Palestinian Land for Treatment of Israeli Waste, December. B'Tselem (2009). The Israeli Information Center for Human Rights in the Occupied Territories. Foul Play. Neglect of Wastewater Treatment in the West Bank, June https://www.btselem.org /publications/summaries/201712_made_in_israel (accessed 15 August 2022).

107 Mbembe, A. (2003). Necropolitics. *Public Culture* 15(3): 11–40.

108 Agamben, Giorgio (1998). *Homo Sacer: Sovereign Power and Bare Life.* Stanford: Stanford University Press.

Conclusion

1 Rasgon, Adam and Kingsley, Patrick (2021). As Palestinians Clamor for Vaccine, Their Leaders Divert Doses to Favored Few. *The New York Times,* 03 March. https://www.nytimes.com/2021/03/03/world/middleeast/ Palestinians-Israel-vaccine-favoritism.html (accessed 14 July 2021).

2 Fanon, Frantz (1994). *A Dying Colonialism.* Boston: Grove Atlantic.

3 Wolfe, P. (2006). Settler-Colonialism and the Elimination of the Native. *Journal of Genocide Research* 8(4): 387–409.

4 Abu Sitta, Salman (2003). Traces of Poison–Israel's Dark History Revealed. *Ahram Weekly,* 27 February–5 March. https://www.plands.org/en/articles -speeches/articles/2003/traces-of-poison%E2%80%93israels-dark-history -revealed (accessed 18 October 2022).

5 Butler, Judith (2020). Capitalism Has Its Limits. *Verso Books,* 30 March. www.versobooks.com/blogs/4603-capitalism-has-its-limits (accessed 17 May 2020).

References

Abdalla, Hisham (2017). Palestinians Protest over PA-Israel Security Ties. *Al-Jazeera*, 14 March.

Abed, Yehia (2020). COVID-19 in the Gaza Strip and the West Bank under the Political Conflict in Palestine. *South Eastern European Journal of Public Health (SEEJPH)* XIV: 1–12. doi: 10.4119/seejph-3543.

Abed Elrazik, Adnan, Amin, Riyad and Davis, Uri (Spring 1978). Problems of Palestinians in Israel, Land, Work, Education. *Journal of Palestine Studies* 7(3): 31–54.

Abu Hatoum, Nayrouz (2021). For 'a no-State Yet to Come': Palestinian Urban Place-Making in Kufr Aqab, Jerusalem. *Environment and Planning E: Nature and Space* 4(1): 85–108.

Abujidi, Nurhan (2009). The Palestinian States of Exception and Agamben. *Contemporary Arab Affairs* 2(2): 272–91.

Abu-Odah, H., Ramazanu, S., Saleh, E., Bayuo, J., Abed, Y. and Salah, M. S. (2021). COVID-19 Pandemic in Hong Kong and Gaza Strip: Lessons Learned from Two Densely Populated Locations in the World. *Osong Public Health Res Perspect* 12(1): 44–50. doi: 10.24171/j.phrp.2021.12.1.07. PMID: 33659154; PMCID: PMC7899229.

Abu-Saad, Ismael (2008). Where Inquiry Ends: The Peer Review Process and Indigenous Standpoints. *American Behavioral Scientist* 51: 1902–18.

Abu-Sada, Caroline (2009). Cultivating Dependence: Palestinian Agriculture under the Israeli Occupation. In Ophir, A., Givoni, M. and Hanafi, S. (eds), *The Power of Inclusive Exclusion: Anatomy of Israeli Rule in the Occupied Palestinian Territories*, 413–34. New York: Zone Books.

Abu-Sittah, Gassan (2020). The Virus, the Settler, and the Siege: Gaza in the Age of Corona. *Journal of Palestine Studies* 49(4): 65–76.

Adalah (2020). The Legal Center for Arab Minority Rights. Israel's Jewish Nation-State Law, 20 December. https://www.adalah.org/en/content/view /9569 (accessed 23 February 2021).

Agamben, Giorgio (1995). We Refugees. Translated by Michael Rocke. *Symposium* 49(2): 114–19. http://www.egs.edu/faculty/agamben/agamben -we-refugees.html (accessed 14 September 2021).

Agamben, Giorgio (1998). *Homo Sacer: Sovereign Power and Bare Life.* Stanford: Stanford University Press.

Agamben, Giorgio (2005). *State of Exception.* Chicago: University of Chicago Press.

Alazzeh, Ala (2015). Seeking Popular Participation: Nostalgia for the First Intifada in the West Bank. *Settler Colonial Studies* 5(3): 251–267.

Alfred, Taiaiake (1999). *Peace, Power, Righteousness: An Indigenous Manifesto.* New York: Oxford University Press.

Alfred, Taiaiake (2005). *Wasáse: Indigenous Pathways of Action and Freedom.* Peterborough: University of Toronto Press.

Al-Hardan, Anaheed (2014). Decolonizing Research on Palestinians: Towards Critical Epistemologies and Research Practices. *Qualitative Inquiry* 20(1): 66, 67.

Al Husseini, Jalal (2010). UNRWA and the Refugees: A Difficult but Lasting Marriage. *Journal of Palestine Studies* 40: 1.

Alkhaldi, Mohammed (2020). Health System's Response to the COVID-19 Pandemic in Conflict Settings: Policy Reflections from Palestine. *Global Public Health* 15(8): 1244–56.

Al Masri, Hani (2016). *Changing the Status Quo: What directions for Palestinians? Is it Possible to Suspend Security Coordination?* Ramallah: The Palestinian Center for Policy and Survey Research (PSR).

Al-Tamimi, Abd Al-Rahman (2021). *Palestinian Water: From Control to Annexation* (Arabic). Ramallah, Palestine: Institute of Palestine Studies.

Al-Shu'aibi, Azmi (2012). Security Sector Reform in the Arab Countries: The Case of Palestine. ARI Thematic Studies: Arab Securitocracies and Security Sector Reform. https://www.arab-reform.net/en/node/580 (accessed 13 May 2019).

Andoni, Lamis (1997). Redefining Oslo: Negotiating the Hebron Protocol. *Journal of Palestine Studies* 25(3): 17–30.

Anton, Glenna (2008). Blind Modernism and Zionist Waterscape The Huleh Drainage Project. *Jerusalem Quarterly* 35: 90.

ARIJ (2012). Kafr 'Aqab Village Profile. Applied Research Institute Jerusalem.

Aruri, Nasser (1999). The Wye Memorandum: Netanyahu's Oslo and Unreciprocal Reciprocity. *Journal of Palestine Studies* 25(2): 17–28.

Ashly, Jaclynn (2018). Palestinians in Kufr Aqab: 'We Live Here Just to Wait'. *Aljazeera*, 07 January. https://www.aljazeera.com/news/2018/1/7/palestinians-in-kufr-aqab-we-live-here-just-to-wait (accessed 18 June 2021).

Association for Civil Rights in Israel (ACRI) (2017). Implications of
Establishing a Separate Local Authority for the Neighborhoods beyond the
Barrier in Jerusalem. Position Paper, November. https://law.acri.org.il/en/
wp-content/uploads/2017/11/Separate-Municiplaity-Position-Paper-1.pdf
(accessed 19 June 2021).

Badarin, Emile (2015). Settler-Colonialist Management of Entrances to the
Native Urban Space in Palestine. *Settler Colonial Studies* 5(3): 226–35.

Badarin, Emile (2016). *Palestinian Political Discourse: Between Exile and
Occupation*. London: Routledge.

BADIL Resource Center for Palestinian Residency & Refugee Rights (2016).
Forced Population transfer: The Case of the Old City of Hebron. Brief,
October 2016. https://www.badil.org/phocadownloadpap/badil-new
/publications/research/working-papers/CaseStudyFPT-Hebron-Brief
-Eng(Oct2016).pdf (accessed 13 June 2021).

Barghouti, Mourid (2004). *I Saw Ramallah*. Translated by Ahdaf Soueif.
London: Bloomsbury Publishing PLC.

Beaumont, Peter (2015). PLO leadership votes to suspend security
cooperation with Israel. *The Guardian*, 5 March. https://www.theguardian.
com/world/2015/mar/05/plo-leadership-votes-to-suspend-security-
cooperation-with-israel (accessed 24 July 2020).

Beaumont, Peter and Holmes, Oliver (2018). US Confirms End to Funding
for UN Palestinian Refugees. *The Guardian*, 31 August. https://www
.theguardian.com/world/2018/aug/31/trump-to-cut-all-us-funding-for
-uns-main-palestinian-refugee-programme (accessed 24 May 2019).

Benvenisti, Meron (1995). *Intimate Enemies: Jews and Arabs in a Shared Land*.
Berkeley: University of California Press.

Benvenisti, Meron (2010). United We Stand: Do Israelis and Palestinians belong
to One Divided Society, or to Two Separate Societies in a Situation of Forced
Proximity as a Result of a Temporary Occupation? *Ha'aretz*, 28 January.

Berda, Yael (2017). *Living Emergency: Israel's Permit Regime in the Occupied
West Bank*. Stanford: Stanford University Press.

Bishara, Marwan (2001). *Palestine/Israel: Peace or Apartheid: Prospects for
Resolving the Conflict*. London: Zed Books.

Bouillon, Markus E. (2004). Gramsci, Political Economy, and the Decline of
the Peace Process. *Critique: Critical Journal of Middle East Studies* 13, no. 3
(Fall): 239–64.

Bouris, Dimitris (2010). The European Union's Role in the Palestinian
Territory after the Oslo Accords: Stillborn State-Building. *Journal of*

Contemporary European Research 6(3): 376–94. http://www.jcer.net/ojs/ index.php/jcer/article/view/205/232 (20 July 2020).

Breaking the Silence (2017). The High Command, Settler Influence on IDF Conduct in the West Bank. https://www.breakingthesilence.org.il/inside/wp -content/uploads/2018/03/THC_Eng_210318.pdf (accessed 28 June 2021).

Breaking the Silence (2018). Occupying Hebron, Soldiers' Testimonies from Hebron 2011–2017, November. https://www.breakingthesilence.org.il/ inside/wp-content/uploads/2018/11/OccupyingHebron-Eng.pdf (accessed 28 June 2021).

B'Tselem (2015). New Restrictions on Movement in Hebron and Environs Disrupt Lives and Constitute Prohibited Collective Punishment. https:// www.btselem.org/freedom_of_movement/20151105_hebron_area

B'Tselem (2017). East Jerusalem, 11 November. https://www.btselem.org/ jerusalem (accessed 18 July 2020).

B'Tselem (2018). The Israeli Information Center for Human Rights in the Occupied Territories Three Israeli Supreme Court Justices Greenlight State to Commit War Crime, 27 May. https://www.btselem.org/communities _facing_expulsion/20180527_supreme_court_greenlights_war_crime_in _khan_al_ahmar (accessed 15 August 2022).

B'Tselem (2019). Playing the Security Card, Israeli Policy in Hebron as a Means to Effect Forcible Transfer of Local Palestinians, September. https:// www.btselem.org/sites/default/files/publications/201909_playing_the _security_card_eng.pdf (accessed 22 June 2021).

B'Tselem (2021). The Israeli Information Center for Human Rights in the Occupied Territories. A Regime of Jewish Supremacy from the Jordan River to the Mediterranean Sea: This is Apartheid, 12 January. https://www .btselem.org/publications/fulltext/202101_this_is_apartheid (accessed 03 May 2021).

Clarno, Andy (2017). *Neoliberal Apartheid: Palestine/Israel and South Africa after 1994*. Chicago and London: University of Chicago Press.

Cook, Jonathan (2018). Is Leaked Document Trump's 'Deal of the Century?' *Middle East Eye*, 9 May. https://www.jonathan-cook.net/2019-05-09/is -leaked-document-trumps-deal-of-the-century/ (accessed 04 May 2020).

Coulthard, Glen S. (2014). *Red Skin, White Masks: Rejecting the Colonial Politics of Recognition*. Minneapolis: University of Minnesota Press.

Daher-Nashif, S. (2021). Colonial Management of Death: To be or not to be Dead in Palestine. *Current Sociology* 69(7): 945–62.

Dajani, Muna, De Leo, Daniela and AlKhalidi, Nora (2013). Planned Informality as a By-Product of the Occupation: The Case of Kufr Aqab Neighborhood in Jerusalem North. *Planum* 26(1): 1–10.

Davis, Angela Y. (2016). *Freedom Is a Constant Struggle: Ferguson, Palestine, and the Foundations of a Movement*. Chicago: Haymarket Books.

Derek, Gregory (2004). *The Colonial Present: Afghanistan, Palestine, Iraq*. Oxford: Blackwell Publishing.

Dunbar-Ortiz, Roxanne (2014). *An Indigenous Peoples' History of the United States*. Boston: Beacon Press.

Dunbar-Ortiz, Roxanne and Gilio-Whitaker, D. (2016). *'All the Real Indians Died Off': And 20 Other Myths about Native Americans*. Boston: Beacon Press.

FACTS Information Committee (1988). *Towards a State of Independence: The Palestinian Uprising, December 1987–August 1988*. http://www.jmcc.org/Documentsandmaps.aspx?id=609 (accessed 07 September 2020).

Falah, Gh. and Flint, C. (2004). Geopolitical Spaces: The Dialectic of Public and Private Spaces in the Palestine–Israel Conflict. *Arab World Geographer* 7: 11–134.

Fanon, Frantz (1963). *The Wretched of the Earth*. New York: Grove Press.

Fanon, Frantz (1967 [1964]). *Toward the African Revolution*. Translated by Haakon Chevalier. New York: Grove Press.

Fanon, Frantz (1994). *A Dying Colonialism*. Boston: Grove Atlantic.

Fanon, Frantz (2008). *Black Skin, White Masks*. London: Pluto Press.

Farsakh, Leila (2008). Independence, Cantons or Bantustans: Whither the Palestinian State? *Middle East Journal* 59, no. 2 (Spring): 238.

Fast, Larissa (2006). Aid in the Pressure Cooker Humanitarian Action in the Occupied Palestinian Territory. *Humanitarian Agenda*, Case Study no. 7. Boston: Feinstein International Center.

Foucault, Michel (1978). *The History of Sexuality*. New York: Vintage.

Foucault, Michel (1990). *The History of Sexuality , Vol. 1, An Introduction*. Translated by Robert Hurley. London: Penguin Books.

Foucault, Michel (1991). *Discipline and Punish: The Birth of a Prison*. London: Penguin.

Foucault, Michel (1995). *Discipline and Punish: The Birth of the Prison*. New York: Vintage Books.

Foucault, Michel (2003a). *Society must be Defended: Lectures at the Collège de France, 1975–76*. New York: Picador.

Foucault, Michel (2003b). *Abnormal. Lectures at the Collége de France 1974–1975.* Translated by Graham Burchell. London and New York: Verso Books.

Ghanim, Honaida (2008). Thanatopolitics: The Case of the Colonial Occupation in Palestine. In *Thinking Palestine*, 65–81. London: Zed Books.

Gisha (2011). Scale of Control: Israel's Continued Responsibility in the Gaza Strip, November. http://gisha.org/UserFiles/File/scaleofcontrol/scaleofcontrol_en.pdf (accessed 11 June 2021).

Gisha (2012). Reader: 'Food Consumption in the Gaza Strip - Red Lines'. https://www.gisha.org/UserFiles/File/publications/redlines/redlines-position-paper-eng.pdf (accessed 07 June 2021).

Gisha (2021). Gaza Up Close, 01 September. https://features.gisha.org/gaza-up-close/ (accessed 08 September 22).

Gramsci, Antonio, Hoare, Quintin and Nowell-Smith, Geoffrey (1971). *Selections from the Prison Notebooks of Antonio Gramsci.* New York: International Publishers.

Grande, S. (2015). *Red Pedagogy: Native American Social and Political Thought.* New York: Rowman & Littlefield.

Greenberg, Joel (1997). Palestinian Census Ignites Controversy over Jerusalem. *The New York Times*, 11 December. https://www.nytimes.com/1997/12/11/world/palestinian-census-ignites-controversy-over-jerusalem.html.

Haddad, Toufic (2016). *Palestine Ltd: Neoliberalism and Nationalism in the Occupied Territories.* London: I.B. Taurus.

Halper, Jeff (2015). *War against the People: Israel, the Palestinians and Global Pacification.* London: Pluto Press.

Halper, Jeff (2021). *Decolonising Israel, Liberating Palestine: Zionism, Settler Colonialism, and the Case for One Democratic State.* London: Pluto Press.

Hamayel, Layaly, Hammoudeh, Doaa and Welchman, Lynn (2017). Reproductive Health and Rights in East Jerusalem: The Effects of Militarisation and Biopolitics on the Experiences of Pregnancy and Birth of Palestinians Living in the Kufr 'Aqab neighbourhood. *Reproductive Health Matters* 25(sup1): 87–95.

Hamdan, Ayat (2020). Silent Displacement in Occupied Palestine: Hebron as a Case Study. Doctoral dissertation, University of Exeter (Unpublished, permission has been granted).

Hammami, Rema (1995). NGOs: The Professionalization of Politics. *Race & Class* 37(2): 51–63.

Hammoudeh, D., Hamayel, L. and Welchman, L. (2016). Beyond the Physicality of Space: East Jerusalem, Kufr 'Aqab, and the Politics of Everyday Suffering. *The Jerusalem Quarterly* 65: 35–60.

Hammoudeh, Weeam, Jabr, Samah, Helbich, Maria and Sousa, C. (2020). On Mental Health Amid COVID-19. *Journal of Palestine Studies* 49(4): 77–90.

HaMoKed and B'Tselem (1997). The Quiet Deportation: Revocation of Residency of East Jerusalem Palestinians. https://www.btselem.org/publications/summaries/199809_quiet_deportation_continues (accessed 21 June 2021).

Hanafi, Sari (2009). Spacio-Cide: Colonial Politics, Invisibility and Rezoning in Palestinian Territory. *Contemporary Arab Affairs* 2(1): 106–21.

Hanafi, Sari, Chaaban, J. and Seyfert, K. (2012). Social Exclusion of Palestinian Refugees in Lebanon: Reflections on the Mechanisms that Cement their Persistent Poverty. *Refugee Survey Quarterly* 31(1): 34–53.

Hanieh, Adam (2008). Palestine in the Middle East: Opposing Neoliberalism and US Power. *MRzine*, 19 July. http://www.monthlyreview.org/mrzine.

Hanieh, Adam (2016). Development as Struggle: Confronting the Reality of Power in Palestine. *Journal of Palestine Studies* 45(4): 32–47.

Hanieh, Adam and Ziadah, R. (2022). Pandemic Effects: COVID-19 and the Crisis of Development in the Middle East. *Development and Change* 53(6): 1308–34.

Hilal, Jamil (1976). Imperialism and Settler colonialism in West Asia: Israel and the Arab Palestinian struggle. *Utafi* 1(1): 51–70.

Hilal, Jamil (2010). *The Pauperization of Women, Men and Children in the West Bank and Gaza Strip*. Birzeit: Institute for Women's Studies, Birzeit University.

Hilal, Jamil (2015). Rethinking Palestine: Settler-Colonialism, Neoliberalism and Individualism in the West Bank and Gaza Strip. *Contemporary Arab Affairs* 8(3): 351–62. doi: 10.1080/17550912.2015.1052226.

Hilal, Jamil, ed. (2020). *Isolation, Separation and Quarantine*. Palestine: Qattan Foundation.

Human Rights Watch (2021). A Threshold Crossed, Israeli Authorities and the Crimes of Apartheid and Persecution. israel_palestine0421_reportcover_8.5x11 (hrw.org). (accessed 15 August 2022).

Ir Amim (n.d.). The Separation Barrier. https://www.ir-amim.org.il/en/issue/separation-barrier (accessed 20 June 2021).

Irfan, A. (2018). Internationalising Palestine: UNRWA and Palestinian Nationalism in the Refugee Camps, 1967–82. Doctoral dissertation, The London School of Economics and Political Science (LSE).

Jabareen, Hassan and Bishara, Suhad (2019). The Jewish Nation-State Law. *Journal of Palestine Studies* 48(2): 43–57.

Jefferis, D. C. (2012). The 'Center of Life Policy': Institutionalizing Statelessness in East Jerusalem. *Jerusalem Quarterly* 93: 94–103.

Jerusalem Media & Communications Centre (JMCC) (1993). *Israeli Military Orders in the Occupied Palestinian West Bank (1967–1992)*. Jerusalem: JMCC.

Joronen, M. (2019). Negotiating Colonial Violence: Spaces of Precarisation in Palestine. *Antipode* 51(3): 838–57.

Journal of Palestine Studies (1997). The Hebron Protocol. *Journal of Palestine Studies* 26(3): 131–45. doi: 10.2307/2538174.

Kaplan, A. (2018). *Our American Israel: The Story of an Entangled Alliance*. Cambridge, MA: Harvard University Press.

Khalidi, Raja and Samour, Sobhi (2011). Neoliberalism as Liberation: The Statehood Programme and the Remaking of the Palestinian National Movement. *Journal of Palestine Studies* XL(2): 6–25.

Khalidi, Rashid (1997). *Palestinian Identity: The Construction of Modern National Consciousness*. New York: Columbia University Press.

Khalidi, Rashid (2013). *Brokers of Deceit: How the US has Undermined Peace in the Middle East*. Boston: Beacon Press.

Khalidi, Rashid I. (1992). Observations on the Right of Return. *Journal of Palestine Studies* 21, no. 2 (Winter): 29.

Khatib, R., Mataria, A., Donaldson, C., Bossert, T., Hunter, D. J., Alsayed, F. and Moatti, J. P. (2009, April 4). The Health-Care System: An Assessment and Reform Agenda. *Lancet* 373(9670): 1207–17. doi: 10.1016/S0140-6736(09)60111-2. Epub 2009 March 4. PMID: 19268349.

Lloyd, David (2012). Settler Colonialism and the State of Exception: The Example of Palestine/Israel. *Settler Colonial Studies* 2(1): 59–80.

Lustick, Ian (2019). *Paradigm Lost: From Two-State Solution to One-State Reality*. Philadelphia: Pennsylvania University Press.

Makdisi, S. (2010). *Palestine Inside Out: An Everyday Occupation*. New York: Norton.

Mallard, A., Pesantes, M. A., Zavaleta-Cortijo, C. and Ward, J. (2021). An Urgent Call to Collect Data Related to COVID-19 and Indigenous Populations Globally. *BMJ Global Health* 6(3): e004655.

Mamdani, Mahmood (2015). Settler Colonialism: Then and Now. *Critical Inquiry* 41(3): 596–614.

Masalha, Nur (1992). *Expulsion of the Palestinians: The Concept of 'Transfer' in Zionist Political Thought, 1882–1948*. Washington, DC: Institute for Palestine Studies.

Masalha, Nur (2002). The Palestinian Nakba: Zionism, 'Transfer' and the 1948 Exodus. *Global Dialogue* 4(Summer): 3.

Massad, Joseph (1996). Zionism's Internal Others: Israel and the Oriental Jews. *Journal of Palestine Studies* 25, no. 4 (Summer): 53–68.

Mbembe, A. (2003). Necropolitics. *Public Culture* 15(3): 11–40.

McNeely, C. A., Barber, B. K., Giacaman, R., Belli, R. F. and Daher, M. (2018). Long-Term Health Consequences of Movement Restrictions for Palestinians, 1987–2011. *American Journal of Public Health* 108(1): 77–83. https://doi.org/10.2105/AJPH.2017.304043.

Medical Aid for Palestinians (MAP) (2022). Delayed, Denied and Deprived: The Collective Punishment of Palestinian Patients in Gaza in the Context of Israel's 15-Year Blockade, June. https://www.map.org.uk/downloads/ map-al-mezan-access-to-health-online.pdf (accessed 15 September 2022).

Melon, Mercedes (2011). Shifting Paradigms, Israel's Enforcement of the Buffer Zone in the Gaza Strip. https://www.alhaq.org/cached_uploads /download/alhaq_files/publications/Shifting-Paradigms.pdf (accessed 15 June 2021).

Memmi, A. (1974). *The Colonizer and the Colonized*. London: Souvenir Press.

Mharib, 'Abd al-Hafiz (1971, March). ālḥmāʿm wālṣqwr fy āsrāyl ['Hawks and Doves' in Israel]. *Shu'un Filastiniyyah* 1: 5–26.

Middle East Monitor (MEMO) (2020). US Provides $500m to Israel under National Covid Relief Bill, 22 December. https://www.middleeastmonitor .com/20201222-us-provides-500m-to-israel-under-national-covid-relief -bill/?fbclid=IwAR37VmJhSuP7HAY4VJ-uisb_9uoMXh_rEnFxLOHxFd 8tbCBMu8y29pscLdM (accessed 23 December 2020).

Morgensen, Scott Lauria (2013). The Biopolitics of Settler Colonialism: Right Here, Right Now. *Settler Colonial Studies* 1(1): 52–76.

Morris, Benny and Kedar, Z. (2022). 'Cast thy bread': Israeli Biological Warfare during the 1948 War. *Middle Eastern Studies*, 59 (4): 1–25.

Muslih, Muhammad (1990). Towards Coexistence: An Analysis of the Resolutions of the Palestine National Council. *Journal of Palestine Studies* 16(4): 3–29.

Nasasra, Mansour (2017). *The Naqab Bedouins: A Century of Politics and Resistance*. New York: Columbia University Press.

Nasasra, Mansour, Richter-Devroe, S., Abu-Rabia-Queder, S. and Ratcliffe, R. (2015). The Naqab Bedouin and Colonialism. *New Perspectives*, 1–32.

Naser-Najjab, Nadia (2020). Palestinian Leadership and the Contemporary Significance of the First Intifada. *Race & Class* 62(2): 61–79.

Naser-Najjab, Nadia and Khatib, Ghassan (2019). The First Intifada, Settler Colonialism and Contemporary Prospects for Collective Resistance. *The Middle East Journal* 73(2): 187–206.

Nasrallah, Elias (2016). *Testimonies on the First Century of Palestine*. Beirut: Dar Al-Farabi.

OCHA (2008). Closure Update: Main Findings and Analysis, 30 April–11 September, Jerusalem, 4–5.

OCHA (2011). East Jerusalem: Key Humanitarian Concerns Special Focus, March. United Nations, OCHA. http://www.ochaopt.org/documents/ocha _opt_jerusalem_report_2011_03_23_web_english.pdf.

OCHA (2013). Humanitarian Monitor Monthly Report, February 2013, 10. Available at: https://www.ochaopt.org/documents/ocha_opt_the _humanitarian_monitor_2013_03_25_english.pdf (accessed 10 June 2021).

OCHA-Relief Web (2021). The Hospital Built by TİKA Reduces the Burden of COVID19 in Gaza, 14 April. The Hospital Built by TİKA Reduces the Burden of COVID19 in Gaza – occupied Palestinian territory | ReliefWeb (accessed 06 May 2021).

Ophir, Adi (2007). There Are No Tortures in Gaza. *South Central Review* 24: 33.

Ophir, Adi, Givoni, M. and Hanafl, S., eds (2009). *The Power of Inclusive Exclusion: Anatomy of Israeli Rule in the Occupied Palestinian Territories*. New York: Zone Books.

Palestinian Central Bureau of Statistics (2020). A Tale of the Statistical Number. Ramallah - Palestine.

Palestinian Central Bureau of Statistics (2021). Jerusalem Statistical Yearbook 2021, No. 23. Ramallah – Palestine.

Pappé, Ilan (2006). *The Ethnic Cleansing of Palestine*. Oxford: Oneworld Publications.

Pappé, Ilan (2013). Revisiting 1967: The False Paradigm of Peace, Partition and Parity. *Settler Colonial Studies* 3(3–4): 341–51.

Pappé, Ilan (2017). *Ten Myths About Israel*. London and New York: Verso Books.

Pappé, Ilan and Chomsky, N. (2015). *On Palestine*. London: Haymarket Books.

Peace to Prosperity Plan (2020, January). Peace-to-Prosperity-0120.pdf (archives.gov) (accessed 07 June 2021).

Peel, W. et al. (1937). Report of the Palestine Royal Commission. UNISPAL. http://unispal.un.org/pdfs/Cmd5479.pdf (accessed 21 June 2014). abbr.: United Nations 1937.

Piterberg, Gabriel (2008). *The Returns of Zionism: Myths, Politics and Scholarship in Israel*. London: Verso Books.

Puar, Jasbir K. (2015). The 'Right' to Maim: Disablement and Inhumanist Biopolitics in Palestine. *Borderlands* 14(1): 8.

Qumsiyeh, Mazin B. (2016). A Critical and Historical Assessment of Boycott, Divestment, and Sanctions (BDS) in Palestine. In Ozerdem, Alpaslan, Thiessen, Chuck and Qassoum, Mufid (eds), *Conflict Transformation and the Palestinians*, chapter 5, 89–113. Florence: Taylor and Francis.

Qurei, Aḥmad (2005). *al-Riwāyah al-Filasṭīnīyah al-kāmilah lil-mufāwaḍāt: min Ūslū ilá Kharīṭat al-ṭarīq*. Vol. 1. Bayrūt: Mu'assasat al-Dirāsāt al-Filasṭīnīyah.

Raz, Avi (2012). *The Bride and the Dowry: Israel, Jordan and the Palestinians in the Aftermath of the June 1967 War*. New Haven: Yale University Press.

Rigby, Andrew (1991). *Living the Intifada*. London: Zed Books.

Rishmawi, Mona (1986). *Planning in Whose Interest? Land Use Planning as a Strategy for Judaization*. Ramallah: Al-Haq Organization.

Rouhana, Nadim and Sabbagh-Khoury, Areej (2015). Settler-Colonial Citizenship: Conceptualizing the Relationship between Israel and Its Palestinian Citizens. *Settler Colonial Studies* 5(3): 41.

Roy, Sara (1995). *The Gaza Strip: The Political Economy of De-Development*. Washington, DC: Institute for Palestinian Studies.

Roy, Sara (1999). De-development Revisited: Palestinian Economy and Society since Oslo. *Journal of Palestine Studies* 28(3): 64–82.

Roy, Sara (2002). Why Peace Failed: An Oslo Autopsy. *Current History* 101(651): 8–16.

Roy, Sara (2004). The Palestinian-Israeli Conflict and Palestinian Socioeconomic Decline: A Place Denied. *International Journal of Politics, Culture, and Society* 17, no. 3 (Spring): 365–403.

Roy, Sara (2011). *Hamas and Civil Society in Gaza: Engaging the Islamist Social Sector*. Princeton and Oxford: Princeton University Press.

Roy, Sara (2012). Reconceptualizing the Israeli-Palestinian Conflict: Key Paradigm Shifts. *Journal of Palestine Studies* 41(3): 71–91.

Roy, Sara (2017). If Israel were Smart. *London Review of Books* 39(12). Available at: https://www.lrb.co.uk/v39/n12/sara-roy/if-israel-were-smart (accessed 07 June 2021).

Sabbagh-Khoury, A. (2021). Tracing Settler Colonialism: A Genealogy of a Paradigm in the Sociology of Knowledge Production in Israel. *Politics & Society*, 50(1): 1–40.

Sa'di, Ahmad H. (2016). *Thorough Surveillance: The Genesis of Israeli Policies of Population Management, Surveillance and Political Control towards the Palestinian Minority.* Manchester: Manchester University Press.

Said, Edward (2001). Introduction. In Said, E. W. and Hitchens, C. (eds), *Blaming the Victims: Spurious Scholarship and the Palestinian Question.* New York: Verso Books.

Salamanca, Omar Jabary (2011). Unplug and Play: Manufacturing Collapse in Gaza. *Human Geography* 4(1): 22–37.

Salamanca, Omar Jabary, Qato, M., Rabie, K. and Samour, S. (2012). Past is Present: Settler Colonialism in Palestine. *Settler Colonial Studies* 2(1): 1–8.

Samour, Sobhi (2020). Covid-19 and the Necroeconomy of Palestinian Labor in Israel. *Journal of Palestine Studies* 49(4): 53–64.

Savir, Uri (1998). *The Process: 1,100 days that Changed the Middle East.* New York: Random House.

Sayegh, Fayez (1965). *Zionist Colonialism in Palestine.* Beirut: Research Center, Palestine Liberation Organization.

Sayegh, Fayez (1979). The Camp David Agreement and the Palestine Problem. *Journal of Palestine Studies* 8(2): 3–40.

Sayegh, Fayes (2012). Zionist Colonialism in Palestine (1965). *Settler Colonial Studies* 2(1): 206–25.

Sayigh, Rosemary (2008). *The Palestinians: From Peasants to Revolutionaries.* London: Bloomsbury Publishing.

Sayigh, Yazid (2009). 'Fixing Broken Windows': Security Sector Reform in Palestine, Lebanon, and Yemen. *Carnegie Papers*, Washington: Carnegie Endowment for International Peace.

Schoeberlein, Jennifer (2019). Transparency International Anti-Corruption Brief. Corruption in the Middle East & North Africa, 10 December. https://www.transparency.org/files/content/pages/2019_GCB_MENA _country_profiles.pdf (accessed 09 August 2021).

Selby, Jan (2005). The Political Economy of the Israeli-Palestinian Peace Process: An Introduction. Paper for Panel on the Political Economy of Conflict Transformation, International Studies Association, Hawaii, 1–5 March, 1–24.

Shalhoub-Kevorkian, Nadera (2015). *Security Theology, Surveillance and the Politics of Fear*. Cambridge Studies in Law and Society, Cambridge: Cambridge University Press.

Sharif, Maher (2020). How Will the World After Corona Be? Institute of Palestine Studies blog, 22 May (Arabic).

Shavit, Ari (2015). *My Promised Land: The Triumph and Tragedy of Israel*. Random House.

Shenhav, Yehouda (1999). The Jews of Iraq, Zionist Ideology, and the Property of the Palestinian Refugees of 1948: An Anomaly of National Accounting. *International Journal of Middle East Studies* 31(4): 605–30.

Shiblak, Abbas (1986). *The Lure of Zion*. London: Al Saqi.

Shlaim, Avi (2000). *The Iron Wall: Israel and the Arab World*. London: Allen Lane, The Penguin Press.

Shohat, Ella (1988). Sephardim in Israel: Zionism from the Standpoint of Its Jewish Victims. *Social Text* 19(20): 1–35.

Simpson, Leanne (2011). *Dancing on Our Turtle's Back: Stories of Nishnaabeg Re-Creation, Resurgence and a New Emergence*. Winnipeg: Arbeiter Ring Press.

Sitta, Abu (2003). Salman. Traces of Poison – Israel's Dark History Revealed. *Ahram Weekly*, 27 February—5 March. https://www.plands.org/en/articles -speeches/articles/2003/traces-of-poison%E2%80%93israels-dark-history -revealed (accessed 18 October 2022).

Smith, Linda Tuhiwai (2012). *Decolonizing Methodologies*. London: Zed Books.

Suárez, Thomas (2017). *State of Terror: How Terrorism Created Modern Israel*. Northampton: Olive Branch Press.

Swisher, Clayton E. (2011). *The Palestine Papers: The End of the Road*. London: Hesperus Press Limited.

Tabner, Isaac T. (2020). Five Ways Coronavirus Lockdowns Increase Inequality. *The Conversation*, 8 April. https://theconversation.com/five -ways-coronavirus-lockdowns-increase-inequality-135767 (accessed 15 August 2022).

Tagari, Ehud and Oppenheimer, Yudith (2015). *Displaced in Their Own City: The Impact of Israeli Policy in East Jerusalem on the Palestinian Neighborhoods of the City beyond the Separation Barrier*. Jerusalem: Ir Amin.

Tamari, Salim (1988). What the Uprising Means. Middle East Report, No. 152. *The Uprising*, 24–30.

Tanous, Izzat (1982). *ālflstynywn māḍ mğyd wmstqbl bāhr*. Beirut: Research Center, Palestine Liberation Organization.

Tartir, Alaa (2015). The Evolution and Reform of Palestinian Security Forces 1993–2013. *Stability: International Journal of Security and Development* 4(1): 1–20.

Tawil-Souri, Helga (2011). Colored Identity: The Politics and Materiality of ID Cards in Palestine/Israel. *Social Text* 29(2): 67–97.

Tawil-Souri, Helga (2012). Digital Occupation: Gaza's High-Tech Enclosure. *Journal of Palestine Studies* 41, no. 2 (Winter): 27–43.

The World Bank (2017). Reconstructing Gaza - Donor Pledges, 12 September. https://www.worldbank.org/en/programs/rebuilding-gaza-donor-pledges (accessed 31 May 2021).

Tibon, Amir (2018). Trump Administration Released Dozens of Millions of Dollars to Support Palestinian Security Forces. *Haartetz*, 2 August. https://www.haaretz.com/us-news/.premium-trump-administration-released-dozens-of-millions-of-dollars-to-pa-1.6340023 (accessed 07 June 2021).

Trouillot, Michel-Rolph (2015). *Silencing the Past: Power and the Production of History*, 2nd revised edn. Boston: Beacon Press.

Tuck, Eve and Yang, K. Yayne (2012). Decolonization is not a Metaphor. *Decolonization: Indigeneity, Education & Society* 1(1): 1–40.

Tufajki, Khalil (2000). Settlements: A Geographic and Demographic Barrier to Peace. *Palestine-Israel Journal, of Political, Economics and Culture* 7(3 and 4): 52–8.

Turner, Mandy (2012). Completing the Circle: Peacebuilding as Colonial Practice in the Occupied Palestinian Territory. *International Peacekeeping* 19(4): 492–507. doi: 10.1080/13533312.2012.709774.

UNICEF (2020). The Rights of Children Amid COVID-19, May. https://www.unicef.org/sop/reports/rights-children-amid-covid-19.

United Nation, General Assembly (2021). Human Rights Council. Forty-Sixth Session 22 February–19 March. Written Statement Submitted by United Nations Watch, a Non-governmental Organization in Special Consultative Status, 01 February. https://www.un.org/unispal/wp-content/uploads/2021/03/AHRC46NGO136_170321.pdf (accessed 09 November 2021).

United Nations Office for the Coordination of Humanitarian Affairs (UN-OCHA Occupied Palestinian Territory) (2014). Occupied Palestinian Territory: Gaza Emergency Situation, September (Online). https://www

.ochaopt.org/sites/default/files/ocha_opt_sitrep_04_09_2014.pdf (accessed 08 June 2020).

United Nations Office for the Coordination of Humanitarian Affairs (OCHA) (2020a). Two Years On: People Injured and Traumatized During 'Great March of Return' Still Struggling, 6 April. https://www.ochaopt.org/content /two-years-people-injured-and-traumatized-during-great-march-return -are-stillstruggling#ftn3 (accessed 20 May 2021).

United Nations Office for the Coordination of Humanitarian Affairs (OCHA) (2020b). Unprotected: Settler Attacks against Palestinians on the Rise Amidst the Outbreak of COVID-19, 22 June. https://www.ochaopt.org /content/unprotected-settler-attacks-against-palestinians-rise-amidst -outbreak-covid-19 (accessed June 2020).

United Nations Office for the Coordination of Humanitarian Affairs (OCHA) (2021). Response to the Escalation in the oPt | Situation Report No. 1, 21–27 May 2021, 27 May. https://www.ochaopt.org/content/response-escalation -opt-situation-report-no-1-21-27-may-2021 (accessed 31 May 2021).

United Nations Relief and Works Agency for Palestine Refugees in the Near East (UNRWA) (2020). UNRWA COVID-19 Appeal, August–December. https://www.unrwa.org/sites/default/files/content/resources /unrwa_covid-19_appeal_august-_december_2020.pdf (accessed 14 March 2021).

Veracini, Lorenzo (2010). *Settler Colonialism: A Theoretical Overview*. Basingstoke: Palgrave Macmillan.

Veracini, Lorenzo (2011). Introducing. *Settler Colonial Studies* 1(1): 1–12.

Wafi, Ali and Ziadeh, Saad eddin (2020). The Necessity for Food Sovereignty in Gaza in the Light of the Corona Pandemic. Palestinian Environmental NGOs Network (PENGON). http://www.pengon.org/uploads/Food %20Sovereignty.pdf (accessed 15 August 2022).

Waziyatawin (2012). Malice Enough in their Hearts and Courage Enough in Ours: Reflections on US Indigenous and Palestinian Experiences under Occupation. *Settler Colonial Studies* 2(1): 172–89.

Weizman, Eyal (2007). *Hollow Land: Israel's Architecture of Occupation*. London: Verso Books.

Winter, Yves (2016). The Siege of Gaza: Spatial Violence, Humanitarian Strategies, and the Biopolitics of Punishment. *Constellations* 23(2): 308–19.

Wolfe, Patrick (1999). *Settler Colonialism and the Transformation of Anthropology: The Politics and Poetics of and Ethnographic Event*. London: Cassell.

Wolfe, Patrick (2006). Settler Colonialism and the Elimination of the Native. *Journal of Genocide Research* 8(4): 388–9.

Yesh Din Figures (2018). Ideologically Motivated Crime by Settlers in Hebron Gets Tailwind from Israeli Authorities, November 2018. https://s3-eu-west-1.amazonaws.com/files.yesh-din.org/Hebron_ENG_Nov18.pdf (accessed 17 August 2022).

Yiftachel, Oren (2009). Creeping Apartheid' in Israel-Palestine. *Middle East Report* 253: 7–15.

Zureik, Elia (2001). Constructing Palestine through Surveillance Practices. *British Journal of Middle Eastern Studies* 28(2): 205–27.

Zureik, Elia (2016). *Israel's Colonial Project in Palestine: Brutal Pursuit.* Abingdon: Routledge.

Index